Perioperative Management of the Patient with Congenital Heart Disease

Edited by

William J. Greeley, MD

Associate Professor of Anesthesiology and Pediatrics
Chief Medical Officer
Duke Children's Hospital
Durham, NC

With 17 contributors

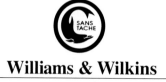

Williams & Wilkins

BALTIMORE • PHILADELPHIA • HONG KONG
LONDON • MUNICH • SYDNEY • TOKYO

A WAVERLY COMPANY

Perioperative Management of the Patient with Congenital Heart Disease

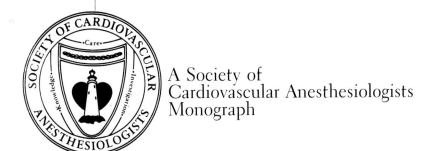

A Society of
Cardiovascular Anesthesiologists
Monograph

Accurate indications, adverse reactions, and dosage schedules for drugs are provided in
this book, but it is possible that they may change. The reader is urged to review the pack-
age information data of the manufacturers of the medications mentioned.

Printed in the United States of America
(ISBN 0-683-18302-8)

96 97 98 99
1 2 3 4 5 6 7 8 9 10

Contributors

Victor C. Baum, MD
Associate Professor
Departments of Anesthesiology
   and Pediatrics
University of Virginia Medical
   Center
Charlottesville, Virginia

Nancy D. Bridges, MD
Director of Pulmonary
   Hypertension and Heart-Lung
   Transplantation Services
Department of Pediatrics
Children's Hospital of
   Philadelphia
University of Pennsylvania
   School of Medicine
Philadelphia, Pennsylvania

Frederick A. Burrows, MD
Associate Professor
Department of Anesthesia
Boston Children's Hospital and
   Harvard Medical School
Boston, Massachusetts

Michael K. Cahalan, MD
Professor
Department of Anesthesia and
   Pediatrics
University of California, San
   Francisco
San Francisco, California

William J. Greeley, MD
Associate Professor of
   Anesthesiology & Pediatrics
Chief Medical Officer
Duke Children's Hospital
Duke University Medical Center
Durham, North Carolina

Dolly D. Hansen, MD
Assistant Professor
Department of Anesthesia
Boston Children's Hospital and
Department of Anesthesia,
   Harvard Medical School
Boston, Massachusetts

David R. Jobes, MD
Professor
Department of Anesthesiology
   and Critical Care Medicine
The Children's Hospital of
   Philadelphia
Philadelphia, Pennsylvania

Didier Journois, MD
Department of Anesthesiology-
   Intensive Care Medicine
Laennec Hospital
Paris, France

Frank H. Kern, MD
Associate Professor
Departments of Anesthesiology
    and Pediatrics
Duke Children's Hospital
Duke University Medical Center
Durham North Carolina

Francis X. McGowan, Jr.,
    MD
Assistant Professor
Department of Anesthesia
Boston Children's Hospital and
    Harvard Medical School
Boston, Massachusetts

Jon N. Meliones, MD
Associate Professor
Departments of Pediatrics and
    Anesthesiology
Duke Children's Hospital
Duke University Medical Center
Durham, North Carolina

Isobel A. Muhiudeen, MD,
    PhD
Associate Professor
Department of Anesthesia and
    Pediatrics
University of California, San
    Francisco
San Francisco, California

Susan C. Nicolson, MD
Associate Professor
Department of Anesthesiology
    and Critical Care Medicine
The Children's Hospital of
    Philadelphia
Philadelphia, Pennsylvania

Philippe Pouard, MD
Department of Anesthesiology-
    Intensive Care Medicine
Laennec Hospital
Paris, France

Norman H. Silverman, MD
Professor
Departments of Pediatrics and
    Radiology
University of California, San
    Francisco
San Francisco, California

Scott R. Schulman, MD
Assistant Professor
Departments of Anesthesiology
    and Pediatrics
Duke Children's Hospital
Duke University Medical Center
Durham, North Carolina

James M. Steven, MD
Assistant Professor
Department of Anesthesiology,
    Critical Care Medicine,
    Pediatrics
The Children's Hospital of
    Philadelphia
Philadelphia, Pennsylvania

Ross M. Ungerleider, MD
Professor
Department of Surgery
Duke Children's Hospital
Duke University Medical Center
Durham, North Carolina

Contents

Preface

Recent developments in cardiovascular surgery for congenital heart disease have resulted in a substantial improvement in patient outcome. Consider for a moment that less than a decade ago there were high mortality rates for certain complex repairs, significant morbidity after repair (central nervous system, heart, lung, etc.), and a significant incidence of residual cardiac defects. Recent improvements in surgical techniques include transatrial repair for tetralogy of Fallot, the arterial switch operation for transposition of the great vessels, and the lateral tunnel procedure with fenestration for Fontan procedures; all of these innovative modifications of surgical technique have directly resulted in a remarkable reduction in mortality for correction of complex lesions. The long-term survival rate for congenital heart surgery is excellent; the 10-year survival rate for common defects such as ventricular septal defects, pulmonic stenosis, atrial septal defects, or coarctation is greater than 90% and greater than 65% for complex lesions such as tetralogy of Fallot, tricuspid atresia, and transposition of the great vessels. In another development, the intraoperative assessment of congenital heart repairs using echocardiography with color flow imaging has decreased the incidence of residual structural defects and has reduced long-term physical disability.

Today cardiopulmonary bypass is much safer, particularly in small infants, due to our improved knowledge of the effects of this technology through systematic investigation and research. The deleterious effects of cardiopulmonary bypass due to such factors as hemodilution and systemic inflammation can be modified using intraoperative hemofiltration. Effective brain protection strategies have led to improvement in neuropsychological dysfunction after cardiac surgery in neonates, infants, and children. The move toward a team concept of perioperative care of these patients, which includes cardiologists, intensivists, anesthesiologists, and surgeons, has been a successful model of interdisciplinary care for many programs in achieving continuous improvement of outcomes through multidisciplinary care and learning. The innovative use of interventional cardiology in the perioperative period is a further demonstration of an interdisciplinary collaboration between surgeon, cardiologist, and anesthesiologist which has yielded improvements in patient outcome in selected repairs. Finally, with the improvement in the health status of these patients, normal adolescence and adult living has been achieved in most cases. Consequently, these patients are requiring anesthesia under less adverse conditions, for noncardiac surgery, for obstetrical deliveries, or for orthopedic procedures, etc.

A monograph of this size cannot provide a comprehensive review of all issues related to anesthesia for congenital heart surgery. In this 9th SCA Monograph, I have attempted to select topics that focus on the most recent developments in surgery for congenital heart disease which have directly led to substantive improvements in patient outcome. In most circumstances, the authors are the original investigators and champicns of the developmental areas in their respective chapters. Because of their specialized expertise, the authors are able to competently present "state-of-the-art" issues and to distill complex topics into succinct, readable, and usable chapters. Where there appear to be gaps in our knowledge, it is my sincere hope that the readers will fill them with new knowledge and findings from their own investigations.

My thanks to the authors for providing an excellent review of their topics and for a job well done. A special thanks also to my mentor and colleague, Jerry Reves, for his support and insights in this endeavor.

WILLIAM J. GREELEY, MD
Associate Professor of Anesthesiology and Pediatrics
Chief Medical Officer
Duke Children's Hospital
Durham, NC

Jon N. Meliones
Frank H. Kern
Scott R. Schulman
Ross M. Ungerleider
William J. Greeley

Pathophysiological Directed Approach to Congenital Heart Disease: a Perioperative Perspective

1

The care of infants and children with congenital heart disease (CHD) has undergone a significant evolution. With improvements in myocardial protection, surgical techniques, and perioperative care, early neonatal repair is now being recommended for the majority of congenital heart lesions.[1-3] Early repair requires a coordinated, multidisciplinary approach to patient care and, as such, requires input from pediatric cardiologists, pediatric cardiac surgeons, pediatric intensivists, pediatric cardiovascular anesthesiologists, perfusionists, specialized nurses, and respiratory therapists. A multidisciplinary approach is necessary in the preoperative period in order to appropriately identify the patient's anatomy and physiology and to determine the correct surgical intervention. A diverse group of health care providers is also essential to assist in performing the surgical procedure and to optimize the patient's postoperative recovery.

The function of the cardiorespiratory system is to provide adequate oxygen delivery in order to meet the metabolical demands and to eliminate the carbon dioxide that is generated.[4-6] Achieving these goals requires a variety of interactions between the cardiovascular and respiratory systems. If the cardiorespiratory system fails to provide adequate oxygen delivery to meet the metabolical needs, anaerobic metabolism occurs which results in acidosis and, ultimately, in organ

Perioperative Management of the Patient with Congenital Heart Disease, edited by William J. Greeley. Williams & Wilkins, Baltimore © 1996.

dysfunction.[4-6] The cornerstone of a multidisciplinary approach to managing cardiac patients is based on the prevention of acidosis and organ dysfunction by providing adequate oxygen delivery. In the perioperative period, the physicians must be acutely aware of the patient's pathophysiology and whether changes in cardiorespiratory interactions are necessary to improve oxygen delivery. In the postoperative period, the physician must understand normal convalescence from cardiac surgery so that abnormal postoperative convalescence can be identified and treated.

The causes for abnormal convalescence can be grouped into three categories: 1) the pathophysiology of the defect prior to surgery and the acute changes in physiology that result from surgery; 2) the presence of residual anatomical defects; and 3) the effects of the "systems" used during repair (e.g., hypothermic cardiopulmonary bypass and/or deep hypothermic circulatory arrest) on organ function. These conditions may result in prolonged convalescence and increased morbidity and mortality.

This chapter is divided into four sections to develop a treatment strategy based on cardiorespiratory physiology. The first section will outline the preoperative management and how stabilization of the patient is achieved prior to surgery. The second section will discuss the methods of recognizing abnormal postoperative convalescence. The third section will address the three causes of abnormal convalescence, including diagnosis and treatment. And, finally, in the fourth section, the management of specific pathophysiological conditions will be presented to demonstrate the multidisciplinary approach.

PREOPERATIVE MANAGEMENT

Tremendous strides in preoperative management have occurred over the past few years and have demonstrated that preoperative stabilization reduces the morbidity and mortality associated with surgery for CHD.[7] The goals of preoperative management are: 1) to stabilize the patient by optimizing oxygen delivery to the tissues, reversing acidosis, and reversing any organ dysfunction that has resulted from decreased oxygen delivery; 2) to provide time to perform an accurate anatomical and physiological diagnosis so that the appropriate surgical procedure(s) can be defined; 3) to prepare the cardiorespiratory system for changes in physiology that may occur after surgery; and 4) to recognize failure of medical management and true surgical emergencies. To understand how one meets these goals, it is helpful to categorize patients into those with acyanotic heart disease and those with cyanotic heart disease. These patients have unique pathophysiological differences necessitating a physiological approach to preoperative management.

Acyanotic Heart Disease

Patients with acyanotic heart disease have normal systemic arterial saturation and no evidence for a right-to-left shunt. There are three categories of patients with acyanotic heart disease: 1) left-to-right shunts (e.g., ventricular septal defect); 2) ventricular inflow-outflow obstructions (e.g., aortic stenosis, pulmonary stenosis); and 3) primary myocardial dysfunction (e.g., cardiomyopathy). The acyanotic patient develops a decrease in oxygen delivery as a result of a reduction in systemic output. The diagnosis of decreased systemic output is supported by the signs and symptoms of decreased oxygen delivery. Clinically, this presents as poor tissue perfusion, decreased capillary refill, hypotension, and tachycardia. Noninvasive testing, including chest x-ray and echocardiography, is helpful in determining the presence of an enlarged heart and myocardial dysfunction. Laboratory tests may demonstrate anaerobic metabolism with the development of acidosis. The therapy for myocardial dysfunction is based on improving systemic output by optimizing preload and contractility while reducing afterload as described in the following sections.

Patients with acyanotic heart disease and increased pulmonary blood flow may develop pulmonary hypertension in the preoperative period. Pulmonary vascular resistance may be elevated immediately after birth.[8,9] Because of the decreased pulmonary blood flow in utero, the pulmonary vessels have a small lumen size at birth. Consequently, these vessels have high pressure and resistance.[8] With the increase in pulmonary blood flow that occurs normally after the first week of life, there is an increase in lumen size and a reduction of pulmonary pressure and resistance. Therefore, some neonates who undergo early cardiac repair may have an increased risk for pulmonary artery hypertension. Attempts to reduce pulmonary artery pressures in the preoperative period may improve oxygen delivery, stabilize the patient prior to surgery, and reduce the risk for pulmonary hypertensive crisis in the postoperative period. An initial preoperative measure to reduce pulmonary hypertension includes the use of increased concentrations of inspired oxygen to improve arterial and alveolar partial pressure of oxygen.[10,11] When ventilation is required, hyperventilation and alkalosis may also help to reduce pulmonary vascular resistance. The treatment strategy for patients with pulmonary hypertension is discussed in a later section (Fig. 1–1).

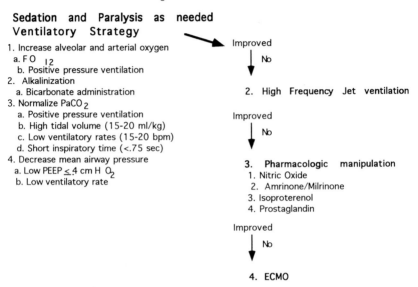

Pulmonary Artery Hypertension

Diagnosis: Decreased oxygen delivery due to pulmonary hypertension and decreased right ventricular cardiac output

Treatment: Decrease right ventricular afterload

Sedation and Paralysis as needed
Ventilatory Strategy

1. Increase alveolar and arterial oxygen
   a. FO_{12}
   b. Positive pressure ventilation
2. Alkalinization
   a. Bicarbonate administration
3. Normalize $PaCO_2$
   a. Positive pressure ventilation
   b. High tidal volume (15-20 ml/kg)
   c. Low ventilatory rates (15-20 bpm)
   d. Short inspiratory time (<.75 sec)
4. Decrease mean airway pressure
   a. Low PEEP $\leq$ 4 cm H O_2
   b. Low ventilatory rate

Improved → No

2. **High Frequency Jet ventilation**

Improved → No

3. **Pharmacologic manipulation**
   1. Nitric Oxide
   2. Amrinone/Milrinone
   3. Isoproterenol
   4. Prostaglandin

Improved → No

4. **ECMO**

FIGURE 1–1. Decision-making algorithm for postoperative patients with pulmonary artery hypertension. Manipulations of pH, FIO_2, and ventilatory mechanics are the most crucial. PEEP, positive end expiratory pressure.

Patients with acyanotic heart disease may also develop pulmonary edema and a reduction in oxygen content due to intrapulmonary shunting (ventilation-perfusion mismatch in the lungs). This develops in lesions associated with increased left atrial pressure which occurs in patients with left ventricular inflow obstruction, diastolic dysfunction of the left ventricle, or increased pulmonary blood flow. These patients will demonstrate an increased respiratory rate, diffuse crackles on chest auscultation, and increased work of breathing. The chest x-ray will demonstrate a congestion pattern. Treatment strategies are directed at increasing oxygen content. These patients will benefit from oxygen administration to overcome the hypoxia and diuretic therapy to reduce the intravascular volume and left atrial pressure. Positive pressure ventilation with positive end expiratory pressures can improve ventilation/perfusion mismatch by opening collapsed alveoli (increase functional residual capacity), increasing tidal volume, and decreasing the work of breathing.[12] Another approach to increasing oxygen content is to increase the hemoglobin. This will increase the oxygen-carrying capacity and will have a secondary benefit of decreasing the intracardiac shunting (by decreasing requirements on cardiac work) in patients with a large left-to-right shunt and is an essential approach to these patients.

Cyanotic Heart Disease

Patients with cyanotic heart disease have a right-to-left shunt and therefore always demonstrate systemic arterial desaturation.[13] These patients do not, however, always have decreased pulmonary blood flow. Patients with cyanotic heart disease are divided into two physiologically distinct groups depending on the role of the ductus arteriosus. These two groups consist of patients with ductal-dependent pulmonary blood flow and, therefore, decreased pulmonary blood flow and patients with ductal-dependent systemic blood flow and, therefore, increased pulmonary blood flow. This grouping allows the development of a physiology-specific approach to preoperative management.

Ductal-Dependent Pulmonary Blood Flow (Decreased Pulmonary Blood Flow)

Patients with ductal-dependent pulmonary blood flow may present with severe hypoxemia and acidosis. This category of patients has a decreased amount of systemic venous blood entering the pulmonary circulation. The obstruction is usually related to an inability of the pulmonary ventricle to deliver blood to the pulmonary circuit. Patients in this group may have obstruction to flow from the pulmonary ventricle either at the outlet (e.g., tetralogy of Fallot [TOF]) or inlet (e.g., tricuspid atresia). The decreased pulmonary blood flow results in a reduction in systemic oxygen saturation, decreased oxygen-carrying capacity, and decreased oxygen delivery. In the initial stages, systemic perfusion may be normal, and the reduction in oxygen delivery is related to a reduction in oxygen-carrying capacity. If oxygen delivery remains inadequate, anaerobic metabolism and myocardial dysfunction develop, which result in a further reduction in oxygen delivery. The end result can be severe hypoxemia and acidosis. Patients with decreased pulmonary blood flow will require a stable form of pulmonary blood flow and a high hemoglobin concentration (>14 mg/dl) in order to maximize oxygen content.

One stable, albeit temporary, form of pulmonary blood flow is the ductus arteriosus. Prostaglandin E_1 has been shown to be a potent dilator of the ductus arteriosus and therefore can provide effective pulmonary blood flow in lesions with decreased flow.[14,15] The institution of prostaglandin E_1 can be life sustaining and provides appropriate time for the reversal of acidosis and organ dysfunction. Prostaglandin E_1 results in an increase in oxygen delivery by increasing oxygen saturation and, therefore, oxygen content. Prostaglandin E_1 is usually infused at a dose of 0.03 to 0.10 μg/kg/minute and may be associated with significant side effects including: tachycardia, hypotension, apnea, and hyperpyrexia. In addition, seizures occur in approximately 5% of patients. The development of apnea requiring mechanical ventilation is of particular concern because this occurs in greater than 40% of cyanotic patients begun on prostaglandin therapy. It should be remembered that prostaglandin E_1 is life sustaining and therefore requires infusion via a functioning central line.

In patients with ductal-dependent pulmonary blood flow, pulmonary blood flow is dependent on three factors: the resistance to flow imposed by the ductus arteriosus, the pulmonary vascular resistance, and the systemic vascular resistance. The resistance to flow imparted by the ductus is usually minimal when infusing prostaglandin E_1, and, therefore, no therapy is directed at manipulating the size of the ductus in patients with decreased arterial saturation despite ductal patency. A reduction in pulmonary vascular resistance and/or increase in systemic vascular resistance can enhance pulmonary blood flow.[8–10] Typically, systemic vascular resistance is not manipulated in the preoperative period for cyanotic patients with ductal-dependent pulmonary blood flow. In patients with decreased arterial saturations despite the presence of a maximally dilated ductus, therapy should be directed at optimizing pulmonary blood flow by lowering pulmonary vascular resistance as outlined below (Fig. 1–2). All patients in this category will require surgical intervention in order to provide a stable source of pulmonary blood flow.

Ductal-Dependent Systemic Blood Flow (Increased Pulmonary Blood Flow)

Patients with ductal-dependent systemic blood flow have increased pulmonary blood flow but decreased systemic blood flow due to obstruction of the aorta which can occur at a variety of locations.[16–18] These patients may have acceptable arterial saturation but develop decreased oxygen delivery as a result of decreased systemic output. This is contrasted to patients with decreased pulmonary blood flow

MANAGEMENT OF SINGLE VENTRICLE PHYSIOLOGY

DECREASED PVR

Diagnosis
 1. Increased sat >85
 2. Decreased mean
   arterial pressure <40

Treatment
 1. Medical
   Dopamine, epinephrine with
 caution due to change in shunt flow
 2. Respiratory
   Increase paCO2 40-55, decrease Ph <7.4
   a. Decrease rate
   b. Decrease Vt 10ml/kg
   c. Increase PEEP 5-10
   d. Add dead space, or CO2 into circuit
   Decrease PaO2
   a. Decrease FiO2 .19

INCREASED PVR

Diagnosis
 1. Decreased sat <75
 2. Increased mean
   arterial pressure

Treatment
 1. Medical
   Amrinone, PGE1
 2. Respiratory
   Decrease paCO2 20-30, Increase Ph>7.55
   a. low rate
   b. High Vt 15-20 cc/kg
   c. decrease PEEP 0-2
   d. HFJV for Paw>10-15
   Increase PaO2
   a. Increase FiO2 1.0

FIGURE 1–2.   Decision-making algorithm for patients with ductal-dependent pulmonary or systemic flow. Unbalanced shunt flow can result in excessive pulmonary or systemic blood flow. Increased pulmonary blood flow results in hyperoxia with systemic hypoperfusion and decreased oxygen delivery. Decreased pulmonary blood flow results in hypoxemia and decreased oxygen content. PEEP, positive end expiratory pressures; PGE_1, prostaglandin E_1.

who develop decreased oxygen delivery due to decreased oxygen content. Patients may present with profound shock due to a dramatic reduction in systemic perfusion and oxygen delivery. Ductal-dependent systemic blood flow occurs in patients with left ventricular outflow obstruction. As in the previous group, prostaglandin E_1 is required. However, in this category of patients prostaglandin E_1 is necessary to allow for systemic perfusion, in contrast to the previous category of patients. Prostaglandin therapy results in stable systemic blood flow and an improvement in oxygen delivery.

Systemic blood flow and, therefore, oxygen delivery, are dependent on the three factors mentioned above: the resistance to flow imposed by the ductus arteriosus, the pulmonary vascular resistance, and the systemic vascular resistance. After maximal dilation of the ductus by prostaglandin E_1 therapy, systemic blood flow can be increased by increasing pulmonary vascular resistance or reducing systemic vascular resistance. Therapy is usually directed at increasing pulmonary vascular resistance (Fig. 1–2) through ventilatory manipulations which include reducing inspired oxygen, preventing hyperventilation, and permitting alveolar hypercapnia. Utilizing prostaglandin therapy and ventilatory manipulations, many of these patients will be stabilized with reversal of the acidosis and organ dysfunction which will result in an improvement in morbidity and mortality.[7,16,18] All patients with these lesions will ultimately require surgical intervention in order to provide a stable form of systemic blood flow.

RECOGNITION OF ABNORMAL POSTOPERATIVE CONVALESCENCE

The recognition of abnormal convalescence is essential in order to optimize patient care. In order to accurately recognize abnormal convalescence, it is necessary to first have an understanding of normal convalescence (Table 1–1). Normal convalescence is dependent on the perioperative pathophysiology and the type of surgical repair involved. Although individual lesions will differ in convalescence, expected plans of care can be developed for the majority of lesions. When evaluating normal convalescence after surgery, estimation of the adequacy of oxygen delivery is essential. This is usually determined by physical examination, ventilatory requirements, and indicators of end-organ function, including: brain (level of consciousness), kidney (urine output), lung (ventilation requirements), heart (cardiac output, filling pressures), and systemic perfusion (pH, lactic acidosis).

Direct measurement of oxygen delivery is now routinely performed in the majority of patients. Cardiac output in most instances should be greater than 2.5 to 3.0 liters/minute/m^2, depending on the extent of the surgical intervention and the postoperative pathophysiology. When cardiac output is not available, mixed venous oxygen saturation trends can provide essential information regarding the adequacy of oxygen delivery. A falling mixed venous oxygen saturation, despite escalating support, indicates abnormal convalescence and the need for aggressive intervention. Another indicator of failing oxygen delivery is the development of metabolical acidosis and/or lactic acidosis. Patients may require intravenous sodium bicarbonate infusion in the immediate postoperative period. However, persistent metabolical acidosis (serum bicarbonate <20 meq/liter) despite bicarbonate administration or administration of high levels of bicarbonate infusion (>3 meq/kg) may indicate inadequate oxygen delivery. Likewise, the sequential evaluation of serum lactate levels provides important information on oxygen delivery. Lactate levels are usually high immediately after surgery but should decrease to <2.0 if oxygen delivery is adequate. Persistent elevations of lactate require evaluation.

TABLE 1–1. INDICATIONS OF NORMAL AND ABNORMAL CONVALESCENCE

Organ System	Normal Convalescence[a]	Abnormal Convalescence
Cardiovascular	Warm extremities, palpable pulses, sinus tachycardia (<25% above normal for age) Blood and central pressures <25% from normal (responsive to interventions) CO >2.5 liters/min/m² ↓ Lactate, ↑ mixed venous saturation Absence of residual defects	Cool extremities, nonpalpable pulses, sinus tachycardia (>25% above n for age) Blood and central pressures > 25% from n (or responsive to supranormal interventions) CO <2.5 liters/min/m² ↑ Lactate, ↓ mixed venous sat Persistent metabolical acidosis ↑ Inotropic support Presence of residual defects
CNS	Sedated, moving extremities	Seizures, delayed awakening, posturing, focal neurological exam, choreoathetosis
Coagulation	Abnormal Pt and Ptt, ↓ platelets, ↓ fibrinogen Chest tube output <10 ml/kg/hr	Bleeding Chest tube output >10 ml/kg/hr
Pulmonary	↓ Compliance Ventilation x 24–48 hr FiO₂ < 0.60 Paw <12 mm Hg	Ventilation >48 hr FiO₂ > 0.60 Paw >12 mm Hg
Renal	Urinary output >1 ml/kg/hr Anuria <24 hr (circulatory arrest patient) Initial hematuria	Urinary output <1 ml/kg/hr Anuria >24 hr (circulatory arrest patient) Prolonged hematuria

[a]CNS, central nervous system; CO, cardiac output; Paw, mean airway pressure.

Urinary output is monitored after cardiac surgery as an indicator of end-organ function and to minimize the toxic side effects of fluid overload (see below). All patients should have at least 1 ml/kg/hour of urinary output within 24 to 48 hours after surgery. Patients without circulatory arrest should have a prompt diuresis and should have >1 ml/kg/hour within the first 24 hours after surgery. Patients who have undergone circulatory arrest may have a period of anuria which should not last >24 to 48 hours.

One of the most important indicators of the state of the cardio-respiratory system is the need for inotropic and ventilatory support. Patients who require extracardiac repair only or placement of an aortopulmonary shunt usually will require little inotropic therapy and minimal ventilation. Patients with simple shunting lesions who require closure (patch or ligature) without valvar involvement include those with atrial septal defects, ventricular septal defects (VSDs), and patent ductus arteriosus. These patients can frequently be extubated in the operating room and require minimal inotropic support. When these procedures are performed in the neonatal period, these patients may require inotropic support of a single agent. Requirements of multiple agents and increasing inotropic requirements signify abnormal convalescence. Patients with more complicated perioperative pathophysiology and those who require circulatory arrest may have a higher inotropic and ventilatory requirement. In the first 24 to 48 hours inotropic support may be generous, and escalation of inotropic support should be anticipated due to myocardial edema/injury. However, failure to respond to moderate increases in inotropic therapy and the need for high levels of inotropic therapy (dopamine/dobutamine >15 μg/kg/minute; amrinone >15 μg/kg/minute; epinephrine >0.1 μg/kg/minute) indicate abnormal convalescence and the need for a thorough investigation.

Respiratory support in the immediate postoperative period should result in a mean airway pressure of <10 mm Hg. A ventilatory requirement resulting in a mean airway pressure >13 to 15 mm Hg is abnormal and requires further investigation as described below. After immediate postoperative stabilization, ventilatory therapy is directed at extubation. One approach is to have patients on pressure support ventilation and to attempt extubation when the spontaneous intermittent ventilation rate is reduced to 5 to 10 beats/minute and the spontaneous tidal volumes are 4 to 6 ml/kg on 5 cm H_2O of pressure support. This should be accomplished in the majority of patients by 72 hours after surgery. If this cannot be accomplished, further diuresis may be required, and the patient must be reevaluated.

In general, patients can be expected to have an inotropic and ventilatory requirement in the first 24 to 48 hours. An increase in inotropic needs can be anticipated. However, failure to respond to increasing support and elevated inotropic needs beyond 48 hours should be considered abnormal. Differentiation of normal vs abnormal convalescence begins in the operating room and extends into the immediate postoperative period.

Operating Room Evaluation

Following repair of a congenital heart defect, the surgeon should attempt to evaluate the quality of that repair before the patient is transferred from the operating room to the intensive care unit. Given the complexity and variety of congenital heart defects currently being repaired, this requires that the operating team inspect the heart for residual intracardiac shunts, areas of stenosis, quality of repaired valve function, flow through and around baffles, and adequacy of ventricular contractility. Several methods for performing this evaluation currently exist and can be utilized in the operating room. The best methods should be easily and quickly performed, provide reliable and easily interpreted information, be sensitive enough to disclose residual problems and specific enough to describe the nature (and location) of these problems. Surgeons frequently use oxygen saturation obtained from various chambers of the heart following discontinuation of cardiopulmonary bypass. This is essentially an intraoperative cardiac catheterization, and a significant "step up" in oxygen saturation may indicate the presence of a residual left-right shunt (e.g., a residual VSD if the right atrial saturation is substantially lower than the saturation in the pulmonary artery). Although this is a simple and easily performed method, it has several limitations. Data may be hard to interpret and can be altered by "streaming" that can produce erroneous information. The other problem with oxygen saturation data is that the information is nonspecific. Even if the test suggests the presence of a significant residual VSD, it cannot demonstrate the location of the problem. In patients who have undergone closure of multiple intracardiac defects, oxygen saturation information cannot localize a residual problem to a specific defect.

Direct pressure measurements can be useful in demonstrating abnormal gradients between chambers or across repaired valves. This information will often guide the operating team to specific areas of residual problems that can often be repaired. This method of assessment may not always lead to a revision of the repair but can be essential in the postoperative period for enabling the team to best care for the patient. An extension of direct measurements obtained in the operating room is the positioning of various intracardiac monitoring lines by the surgeon prior to closing the patient's chest. A right atrial pulmonary artery and left atrial line are usually easily placed by the surgeon and along with a superior vena cava line (usually placed by the anesthesiologist) can continue to provide important information that facilitates patient care in the intensive care unit (ICU) setting. Occasionally, a right or left atrial line will demonstrate prominent V waves suggestive of AV valve insufficiency. Pulmonary artery pressures can be an important parameter to follow after repair of certain defects (e.g., truncus arteriosus, total anomalous pulmonary venous return) and may demonstrate the need for specific ventilator management strategies.

In recent years several groups have reported the use of intraoperative echocardiography to evaluate repair of congenital heart defects.[19-23] Once learned, this method has extraordinary sensitivity and specificity for postrepair problems.[24,25] Intraoperative echocardiography can be performed by anesthesiologists and cardiologists using a transesophageal transducer or by the surgeon using an epicardial transducer.[20,25,26] With the use of intraoperative echocardiography, it is unusual for a patient to be returned to the ICU with a significant, repairable residual defect following congenital heart surgery. This means that the intensive care staff will have a better idea of how to care for the patient, and it is less likely that the patient will require cardiac catheterization and/or return to the operating room in the immediate postoperative period.

Intensive Care Unit Evaluation

The recognition of abnormal convalescence also takes place postoperatively in the ICU by utilizing the extensive monitoring available. Monitoring should be directed at determining whether the goals of the cardiorespiratory system are met in the postoperative period. A variety of approaches has been proposed for monitoring depending upon institutional preferences. Our approach consists of a combination of invasive and noninvasive monitoring to assess oxygen delivery, the physiological state of the patient, and end-organ function. This section will delineate the role of invasive monitoring, laboratory testing, echocardiographic evaluation, and cardiac catheterization in evaluating abnormal convalescence.

Noninvasive Monitoring

Noninvasive monitoring is an important adjunct in assessing the postoperative patient. Noninvasive monitoring includes pulse oximetry and surface electrocardiogram (ECG) monitoring. The surface ECG provides information on heart rate and rhythm. Pulse oximetry plays a crucial role in evaluating patients in the postoperative period, by continuously displaying the patient's arterial oxygen saturation.[13,23,27-29] This can provide important insight into oxygen content and oxygen delivery, as well as information regarding the respiratory system. A fall in arterial oxygen saturation may be the first indication of worsening lung function, accidental extubations, failure of the mechanical ventilator, or a decrease in cardiac output. Because of the potential sensitivity of pulse oximetry for reflecting important acute alterations in the patient's condition, any changes in oxygen saturation should be vigorously investigated.

Invasive Monitoring

Before invasive monitoring is begun in a pediatric patient the risk to benefit ratio for catheter placement should be determined. The risks associated with catheter placement may be higher in neonatal and pediatric patients compared to adults due to the small size of the patients and vessels being cannulated. Percutaneous central venous catheterization is not as easily performed in small infants and can result in inappropriate location of the catheter in the extravascular space. Placement of central venous lines in neonates and small infants can also be time consuming and stressful to the marginal patient, thereby making them unstable. Prolonged cannulation of a vessel can increase the risk of infection or vessel thrombosis. The benefits of catheter placement depend upon the site and type of catheter to be placed. In order to understand the indications for catheter placement it is essential to first understand what information can be derived from blood sampling and pressure data obtained from this invasive monitoring.

Vascular catheters are commonly placed in the operating room and include central venous catheters, right atrial catheters, left atrial catheters, pulmonary artery catheters, and arterial catheters. Central venous or right atrial catheters provide right-sided filling pressures, as well as information about right-sided atrial valve function. Furthermore, they enable indirect assessments of cardiac output by providing systemic venous oxygen saturation.[30] They also provide an excellent site for infusion of pharmacological agents. Because of their relative safety and extraordinary utility, most cardiac surgery patients will have a central venous/right atrial line. There are no contraindications for central venous or right atrial catheterization. Central venous catheterization can be obtained by percutaneous cannulation of the internal jugular vein or by placing the catheter directly into the right atrial appendage at the time of surgery. Percutaneous placement usually requires a 5-cm double-lumen catheter in patients less than 6 months of age. Intracardiac catheters placed by the surgeon at the end of the operation should be well secured to the skin to help prevent them from being inadvertently pulled back into the pleural (mediastinal) space during the postoperative period.[31] Left atrial catheterization provides data on pressures in the left side of the heart, mitral valve function, and presence of right-to-left shunting in the lung. The indications for left atrial catheter placement consist of patients with abnormal mitral valve function, patients with abnormalities of left ventricular diastolic and/or systolic function, and patients with abnormal lung parenchyma. Left atrial catheter placement carries the additional risk of introduction of air to the systemic arterial circulation. This can be kept to a minimum by careful treatment of these lines and appropriate education of the personnel using them. The recent introduction of intraoperative echocardiography has resulted in a more selective use of left atrial lines.[26]

Pulmonary artery catheterization provides information on pulmonary pressures, pulmonary artery saturation, and cardiac output measurements.[31,32] Indications include patients who are at risk for pulmonary hypertension, residual left-to-right shunts, and decreased cardiac output. Pulmonary artery catheters should be utilized in patients whose postoperative pulmonary artery pressures is greater than one-half the systemic arterial pressure and in patients who are at a high risk for pulmonary artery hypertension. Patients who preoperatively have large left-to-right shunts, such as an atrioventricular septal defect, or patients with obstruction at either the pulmonary venous or mitral valve level, usually will require a pulmonary artery catheter (PAC). PACs are placed during surgery through the right ventricular outflow tract and advanced into the main pulmonary artery. Contraindications for PAC placement consist of a large right ventricular outflow tract patch or any anatomical condition which will not allow placement of the catheter through a muscle bundle.

Arterial catheterization is required in all patients who have undergone surgery for congenital heart disease. Arterial catheterization allows repeated measurements of blood gases, electrolytes, calcium, glucose, lactic acid, hematocrit, and liver function studies. In addition, continuous monitoring of blood pressure is provided. Arterial catheters can be readily placed in either the radial, tibial, ulnar, or femoral arteries.

Physical Examination

Clinical assessment is an important adjunct in the evaluation of abnormal convalescence and should be integrated with invasive and noninvasive tests to appropriately determine the status of the cardiorespiratory system. Although a vital part of patient assessment, physical examination remains the least quantifiable and most subjective measure. Physical examination provides a direct assessment of the cardiorespiratory system by auscultation of heart and breath sounds and measurements of tissue perfusion. Assessment of tissue perfusion is performed by examining distal extremity temperature, capillary refill, and peripheral pulses. A prolongation of capillary refill greater than 3 to 4 seconds indicates poor systemic perfusion.

Laboratory Evaluation

Serial evaluation of specific laboratory values are necessary after surgery and include: blood gases, electrolytes, ionized calcium, glucose, lactic acid, hematocrit, and liver function studies. Frequent arterial blood gases are essential in the postoperative period because they provide important information on oxygen delivery and carbon dioxide removal. Evaluation of oxygenation, ventilation, and tissue perfusion is determined by monitoring bicarbonate and base deficits.[33] Frequent monitoring of the ionized calcium level may be necessary in the postoperative period, especially in newborns and infants.[34,35] Infants and newborns are susceptible to changes in ionized calcium levels because the immature heart is more dependent on circulating calcium levels for effective contractility, which is, in part, due to the lack of a well-developed intracellular transport system for calcium. Therefore, adequate circulating ionized calcium levels are essential in maintaining myocardial function. A reduction in ionized calcium may occur in the early postoperative period because of the transfusion of citrate and albumin contained in blood products that bind calcium.[36] It should be noted that total calcium levels do not accurately correlate with ionized calcium levels after cardiopulmonary bypass.[36] This is related to the rapid fluid shifts that occur in the early postoperative period. We recommend measurement of ionized calcium levels every 6 hours for the first 24 to 48 hours after cardiopulmonary bypass. Several groups recommend hourly calcium infusions in neonates and young infants following cardiac repair (e.g., calcium gluconate, 10 mg/kg/hour for 24 to 48 hours) in order to protect against dangerous depressions in ionized calcium levels.

The patient's hematocrit is measured in the postoperative period as an indicator of ongoing bleeding or hemoconcentration. In the early postoperative period, hemoconcentration frequently results from extravasation of fluid into the extravascular space, indicating an ongoing capillary leak. In neonates and infants, extravascular water accumulation occurs more frequently than in adults. Therefore, measuring the hematocrit provides an excellent method for evaluating the extent of this hemoconcentration (e.g., elevations of the hematocrit, in the absence of ongoing blood transfusion, reflect third space fluid loss that must be replaced to maintain hemodynamic stability).[37,38]

The goal for the cardiorespiratory system is to provide adequate oxygen delivery to prevent anaerobic metabolism. Laboratory monitoring of the patient's acid/base status and the development of lactic acid production are important methods of monitoring oxygen delivery and the oxygen supply to demand ratio. Lactic acid levels are usually quite high, 6 to 10 (units) after circulatory arrest and deep hypothermic cardiopulmonary bypass. As tissue perfusion improves, lactic acid levels may decrease rapidly in the ICU. Persistent elevation of lactic acid levels or rising lactic acid levels indicate poor oxygen delivery and/or ongoing organ dysfunction and should initiate a vigorous investigation. Lactic acid levels are often an excellent indicator of the patient's cardiac output, indicating adequacy of end-organ perfusion, and this trend is important to follow during the convalescent period.

Echocardiography

Echocardiography with Doppler color flow imaging is an important tool in the perioperative assessment of patients. Echo-Doppler provides noninvasive information about the anatomy and physiology of the patient and should, therefore, be used liberally in the postoperative period.[16,39–43] The morbidity/mortality associated with congenital heart surgery is directly dependent on the structural integrity of the repair, and potentially treatable defects should be evaluated early in the postoperative period utilizing echocardiography.[44] Echo-Doppler evaluation in the postoperative period can provide interrogation on the surgical repair (presence of residual shunts, valve stenosis/regurgitation, prosthetic valve/conduit function, shunt patency), assessment of ventricular function, and evaluation for tamponade and/or effusions. The limitations of transthoracic echocardiography in the postoperative period include the lack of adequate imaging windows and the presence of lung hyperexpansion and interference from positive pressure ventilation. However, transesophageal echocardiography may be helpful in expanding the use of echocardiography.[23]

Cardiac catheterization is an important adjunct in evaluating abnormal convalescence and is frequently utilized for the diagnosis of residual disease after surgery for congenital heart disease. Cardiac catheterization should be performed in any patient where abnormal convalescence has occurred, and echocardiography does not identify the precise pathophysiological abnormality. An exciting new area in the field of cardiac catheterization is the use of interventional cardiac catheterization to treat residual disease (closing residual shunts or dilating areas of stenosis).[45]

CAUSES OF ABNORMAL CONVALESCENCE

Pathophysiology Prior to Surgery and the Response to Changes in Physiology as a Result of Surgery

The pathophysiological state of the patient prior to surgery may cause abnormalities in the cardiorespiratory system and predispose patients to abnormal convalescence. A variety of conditions may result in pathophysiology in the preoperative period which prolong postoperative recovery. In addition, changes in physiology that occur as a result of surgery or an abnormal response to these changes may contribute to the development of abnormal convalescence. The physiological changes that can occur consist of a reduction or increase in preload and a reduction or increase in afterload to the right or left ventricle. As a result of these changes in physiology, there are three primary pathophysiological disturbances that occur in the postoperative period that lead to abnormal convalescence: left ventricular dysfunction, right ventricular dysfunction, and pulmonary hypertension. These disturbances will be discussed separately.

Left Ventricular Dysfunction

After surgery for congenital heart disease, left ventricular dysfunction may occur.[30,46–52] Left ventricular dysfunction is more easily diagnosed and treated than right ventricular dysfunction but is less frequently observed in pediatric patients. The etiology of postoperative left ventricular dysfunction is usually multifactorial and includes the preoperative condition of the myocardium (left ventricular hypertrophy, left ventricular systolic/diastolic dysfunction), response to alterations in the loading conditions on the left ventricle (increase/decrease in afterload/preload), and the effects of deep hypothermia and/or circulatory arrest (myocardial ischemia) on left ventricular myocardial performance. Left ventricular dysfunction should be considered a cause for prolonged convalescence in any patient with suddenly increased afterload to the left ventricle (e.g., VSD closure, arterial switch for transposition of the great arteries [TGA]) or in any patient with prolonged periods of myocardial ischemia during repair.

The diagnosis of left ventricular dysfunction is based on noninvasive and invasive evaluation. Noninvasive evaluation consists of physical exam, systemic oxygen saturation, chest x-ray, and echo-Doppler. The physical exam will demonstrate evidence for decreased oxygen delivery on the basis of decreased cardiac output. These patients may have tachycardia, hypotension, and poor distal perfusion, as demonstrated by decreased pulses and decreased capillary refill.

The pulse oximetry measurements may be decreased or unattainable due to the inadequate distal perfusion. The chest x-ray will demonstrate cardiomegaly and passive congestion of the respiratory system. Echo-Doppler is valuable in evaluating potentially treatable causes for left ventricular dysfunction and for following the patient's response to interventions. Echo-Doppler may demonstrate ventricular distention, decreased fractional shortening, decreased ejection fraction, and increased end-systolic volume. Invasive testing can also provide information about the presence of left ventricular dysfunction. Invasive catheters placed at the completion of surgery will reveal an increase in left-sided diastolic pressures, decreased mixed venous saturation, and decreased cardiac output. Laboratory testing will demonstrate evidence for a metabolic acidosis and lactic acidosis. When passive congestion of the respiratory system develops, patients are at risk for the development of ventilation-perfusion mismatch with resultant hypoxemia and respiratory acidosis. Patients with significant left ventricular dysfunction will develop end-organ dysfunction as indicated by a reduction in urinary output.

Patients with evidence for decreased cardiac output with or without concomitant acidosis and organ dysfunction will require vigorous investigation into the cause of the dysfunction and the institution of appropriate interventions to support the patient. The treatment is based on the understanding that left ventricular dysfunction results in decreased cardiac output and decreased oxygen delivery (Fig. 1–3). Since cardiac output is a function of heart rate and stroke volume, optimizing these variables will result in an improvement in cardiac output. Left ventricular stroke volume can be modulated by changes in preload, inotropy, and afterload.[62,69–77] Therefore, the management of left ventricular dysfunction requires optimizing the patient's heart rate, preload, inotropic status, and afterload. Patients with low heart rates and neonatal patients with left ventricular dysfunction may increase oxygen delivery by increasing the heart rate. It should be remembered, however, that coronary blood flow to the left ventricle occurs during diastole.[78] An increase in heart rate results in a reduction of diastolic filling time and can reduce left ventricular myocardial blood flow, especially at fast heart rates (>190 beats/min). Therefore, one should manipulate the heart rate cautiously in patients with left ventricular dysfunction. Patients who demonstrate a relative bradycardia will benefit from an increase in heart rate. However, in infants with tachycardia (rates >180 to 200 beats/min), increasing the heart rate may result in an unfavorable supply to demand ratio and should be done cautiously.

Left ventricular stroke volume can be modulated by changes in preload or left ventricular end-diastolic volume. As previously stated,

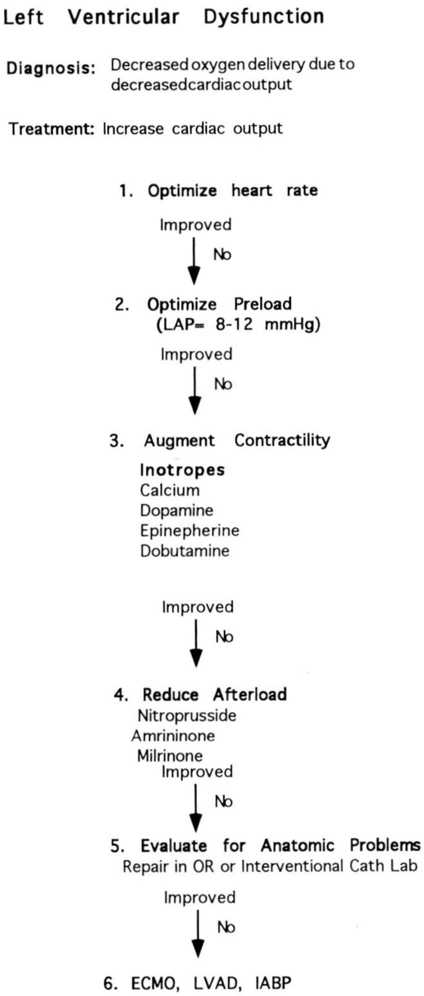

Left Ventricular Dysfunction

Diagnosis: Decreased oxygen delivery due to decreased cardiac output

Treatment: Increase cardiac output

1. Optimize heart rate

   Improved

   ↓ No

2. Optimize Preload
   (LAP= 8-12 mmHg)

   Improved

   ↓ No

3. Augment Contractility

   Inotropes
   Calcium
   Dopamine
   Epinepherine
   Dobutamine

   Improved

   ↓ No

4. Reduce Afterload
   Nitroprusside
   Amrininone
   Milrinone
   Improved

   ↓ No

5. Evaluate for Anatomic Problems
   Repair in OR or Interventional Cath Lab

   Improved

   ↓ No

6. ECMO, LVAD, IABP

FIGURE 1-3. Decision-making algorithm in postoperative patients with left ventricular dysfunction. Oxygen delivery is optimized by manipulating preload, inotrope, and afterload. ECMO, extracorporeal membrane oxygenation; IABP, intraaortic balloon pump; LVAD, left ventricular assist device.

neonates have limited preload recruitable stroke volume above a left ventricular filling pressure of 10 mm Hg.[61,62] Patients with left-sided filling pressures below 10 mm Hg may benefit by increasing the left ventricular end-diastolic volume through volume infusion. Once preload is optimized, increasing the inotropic state of the left ventricle becomes the primary therapy for improving cardiac output.

Alterations in the inotropic state of the left ventricle can be performed by altering circulating calcium levels and administering inotropic agents. Calcium supplementation plays an essential role in augmenting left ventricular function in pediatric patients.[34,73] The underdeveloped sarcoplasmic reticular system in the neonatal myocardium causes the heart to be more dependent on extracellular calcium concentration than the adult myocardium. Since intracellular calcium plays a central role in myocardial contractility in neonates, normal or even elevated blood levels of ionized calcium may be necessary to augment stroke volume. Calcium resuscitation in the postoperative period has fallen into some disfavor in adult patients secondary to the concerns of reperfusion injury. However, calcium supplementation remains an essential component of the management strategy in pediatric patients. Wide fluctuations in ionized calcium levels may occur in the perioperative period, and routine monitoring of ionized calcium levels is essential.

Augmenting the force of ventricular contraction by inotropic agents can result in a significant improvement in cardiac output and oxygen delivery. Vasoactive agents may have different effects in pediatric patients than adult patients, and an understanding of the pediatric patient's response to vasoactive agents is essential. Dopamine is an endogenous catecholamine and is a commonly used vasoactive agent in the perioperative period. Dopamine causes a dose-dependent stimulation of dopaminergic receptors, β_1-receptors and α_2-receptors.[57,69-72] Dopamine augments cardiac contractility through direct stimulation of β_1-receptors in the heart and by inducing norepinephrine release at the presynaptic terminal, which results in stimulation of the β-receptors.[70] Dopamine also has the unique property of binding to dopaminergic receptors that are present in the renal medulla, brain, gut, and coronary bed. Stimulation of dopaminergic receptors results in increased perfusion to these tissue beds. At higher doses, dopamine can result in stimulation of α_2-receptors that are present in the peripheral vascular system. Stimulation of these receptors results in peripheral vasoconstriction. In adult patients, the vasoactive effects of dopamine are dose dependent, and an infusion of dopamine <5 µg/kg/minute will result in dopaminergic stimulation, 5 to 10 µg/kg/minute, β_1 stimulation with augmentation of stroke volume, and >10 to 15 α_1 stimulation. Several studies have been performed in children which suggest that the dose-dependent effects of dopamine are age specific.[69,71,79] In neonates, dopamine increases cardiac output, primarily by increasing heart rate. Neonates have an immature β_1 response, but a mature α_2 response, and may have an increase in blood pressure due to an increase in systemic vascular resistance. Nonetheless, neonates and infants respond favorably to dopamine infusion with increases in oxygen delivery, reversal of acidosis, and end-organ dysfunction. Dopamine is usually begun in neonates and pediatric patients at a dose of 5 to 15 μg/kg/minute and titrated by using noninvasive and invasive measures of cardiac output.

Dobutamine is a vasoactive agent that may augment stroke volume by increasing the force of ventricle contraction. Dobutamine, has primarily β_1 and β_2 effects. As such, it can lead to an increase in force of contraction and peripheral vasodilatation.[75] The advantage of dobutamine over dopamine is the lack of α_2 stimulation. However, in neonatal and pediatric patients the peripheral β_2 effects may predominate, yielding a mild peripheral vasodilatation and little augmentation of ventricular contraction. The efficacy of dobutamine appears to be reduced in immature animals as a result of the reduced β-receptor stimulation and higher levels of circulating catecholamines in newborns.[72] Side effects from dobutamine use include tachyarrythymias due to the structural similarities of dobutamine to isoproterenol. Dobutamine is usually begun at doses of 5 to 10 μg/kg/minute and titrated similarly to dopamine.

Epinephrine is a potent endogenous catecholamine that is useful in the postoperative period. Infusion of epinephrine results in dose-dependent α, β_1, and β_2 stimulation.[75] Epinephrine infused at low doses (0.03 to 0.1 μg/kg/min) will primarily result in β stimulation, with an increase in force of contraction and augmentation of cardiac output. Intermediate doses of epinephrine, 0.1 to 0.2 μg/kg, result in mixed α- and β-receptor stimulation and mixed hemodynamic effects. At doses of epinephrine above 0.2 μg/kg/minute, the predominate effect is α stimulation and peripheral vasoconstriction. The potent effects and side effects result in epinephrine rarely being instituted as a first line agent. However, it is useful in patients with left ventricular dysfunction that remains refractory to dobutamine or dopamine and is usually initiated at 0.03 μg/kg/minute and titrated to effect.

Amrinone is a phosphodiesterase inhibitor which can result in increased inotropy and decreased afterload.[76,80–82] Inhibition of phosphodiesterase results in a decreased breakdown of cyclic AMP and increased calcium available in the cell. The increased calcium in the myocardium results in increased force of contraction, whereas in the peripheral vasculature the increased calcium results in vasodilatation. Studies of the inotropic effects of amrinone in immature animals have yielded contradictory results: Amrinone is a potent vasodilator in immature animals, and the differences in the results of these studies may be in part due to differences in the left ventricular end-diastolic volume of the animals at the time of measurement. The beneficial use of amrinone in patients after surgery for TGA has recently been demonstrated.[82] Amrinone has a long half-life, exceeding 15 hours in some patients, and therefore requires intravenous loading. Pharmacological studies suggest that loading doses for children are twice the recommended adult dosage and should be in the range of 2 to 4 mg/kg.[77] Higher loading doses have been associated with profound systemic vasodilatation and a reduction in cardiac output resulting from a reduction in left ventricular end-diastolic volume. We, therefore, recommend a loading dose of 2 to 3 mg/kg over a 20 to 30-minute period with particular attention to changes in the patient's preload. If preload reduction occurs, as demonstrated by a decrease in filling pressures, volume resuscitation to the patient's previous preload level should be accomplished. Amrinone is infused at a dose of 5 to 10 μg/kg/minute and is especially useful in patients with decreased left ventricular systolic function and increased left ventricular afterload. The development of thrombocytopenia may necessitate the termination of the infusion. Because of the long half-life, milrinone, a phosphodiesterase with a shorter half-life, may replace the use of amrinone in infants and children.

Oxygen delivery can be improved in patients with left ventricular dysfunction by reducing the force opposing left ventricular ejection (afterload). Afterload reduction can be accomplished by the infusion of amrinone or nitroprusside. Nitroprusside is a nitrate that provides direct systemic and pulmonary artery vasodilatation. By reducing afterload and augmenting cardiac output, nitroprusside will result in an increase in cardiac output and oxygen delivery. The half-life of nitroprusside is extremely short and therefore allows a rapid assessment of whether a patient will benefit from afterload reduction while allowing rapid elimination of the drug in patients who develop side effects. Nitroprusside is begun at infusion rates of 1 μg/kg/minute and titrated to effect. Side effects that should be carefully monitored include excessive vasodilatation and nitrate toxicity.

Cardiorespiratory interactions should be evaluated in the postoperative period and directed at optimizing left ventricular function.[33,83–86] These interactions are especially significant in patients with injured myocardium because small changes in ventilatory manipulations can cause a significant change in the cardiorespiratory system. In patients with left ventricular dysfunction we recommend a ventilatory strategy that is designed to optimize left ventricular function (Fig. 1–3). To develop a ventilatory strategy that is specific for patients with left ventricular dysfunction, it is necessary to understand how changes in respiratory physiology alter left ventricular function. An increase in positive end expiratory pressure (PEEP) or mean airway pressure results in a reduction of left ventricular end-diastolic volume and can lead to a decrease in cardiac output.[12,87] Therefore, the ventilatory strategy for patients with left ventricular dysfunction consists of reducing mean airway pressure as low as possible to permit appropriate filling of the ventricle. We recommend the use of high tidal volumes (20 ml/kg) to allow for a "pulmonary pump" effect and augmentation of left-sided blood flow.[88,89] To accomplish this while maintaining mean airway pressure as low as possible, we recommend low ventilatory rates (15 to 20 beats/min) and a short inspiratory time. If patients with left ventricular dysfunction develop pulmonary edema and decreased systemic oxygen saturation, oxygen content may fall, and oxygen delivery will be further compromised. In these instances, the hemoglobin is maintained at a high level, and a higher level of inspired oxygen is initiated. Positive end expiratory pressure may also be necessary to improve oxygenation but should be carefully titrated to ensure enhanced oxygen delivery.

Mechanical support for pediatric patients with a failing left ventricle consists of the use of a variety of devices including an intraaortic balloon pump counterpulsation (IABP), extracorporeal membrane oxygenation, or a left ventricular assist device.[90-95] A complete description of these devices is beyond the scope of this section. Several reviews are provided for the interested reader.[90-95]

Right Ventricular Dysfunction

Right ventricular dysfunction is frequently encountered in infants and children in the postoperative period.[96,97] The majority of these patients will have preexisting cardiac conditions which increase the risk for the development of right ventricular dysfunction. In addition, the changes in physiology that occur as a result of surgery may result in the development of right ventricular dysfunction. Right ventricular dysfunction should be considered as a cause for prolonged convalescence in any patient in whom a right ventricular incision has been used for the repair (e.g., repair of TOF with a transannular patch, transventricular closure of VSD) or in whom the right ventricle was abnormal prior to repair (e.g., TOF, double-outlet right ventricle, pulmonary stenosis, etc.).[58,98,99] Furthermore, it should be expected in any patient whose right ventricle remains volume-loaded following surgery (e.g., first-stage palliation for hypoplastic left heart syndrome).

The diagnosis of right ventricular dysfunction is supported by noninvasive assessment and invasive testing. These patients have evidence of decreased oxygen delivery and increased right-sided filling pressures. Right ventricular dysfunction leads to a decrease in cardiac output because of ventricular interdependence where the left ventricle can only eject the portion of blood that is presented to it by the right ventricle.[100] As a result, decreased cardiac output occurs which is manifest as hypotension, tachycardia, poor tissue perfusion, and prolonged capillary refill. The increased right-sided filling pressure that occurs with right ventricular dysfunction will also cause hepatic congestion. Echocardiography will demonstrate decreased right ventricular shortening and abnormal compliance. Invasive monitoring is diagnostic and demonstrates increased right-sided filling pressures, decreased systemic venous saturation, and decreased cardiac output. Systemic arterial desaturation may occur due to right-to-left shunting at the atrial level in patients with RV dysfunction and a patent foramen ovale or residual shunt following surgery.[27,28]

The treatment of right ventricular dysfunction is directed at improving oxygen delivery using a similar approach as outlined for patients' left ventricular dysfunction (Fig. 1–4). Pharmacological and ventilatory manipulations are directed at increasing right ventricular cardiac output by optimizing preload, inotropy, and afterload.[58,96,97] The right ventricle is less sensitive to conventional inotropes, and therefore preload and afterload are more commonly manipulated to augment cardiac output. Excessive volume overloading, however, needs to be prevented because this can result in tricuspid insufficiency and decreasing right ventricular cardiac output. In general, central venous pressures >12 to 14 mm Hg are poorly tolerated in neonates and infants with right ventricular dysfunction inasmuchas this leads to venous hypertension and capillary leak.[101]

Institution of a positive inotropic agent can result in improved right ventricular cardiac output, coronary flow, and oxygen delivery. The right ventricular myocardium is less sensitive to inotropic agents and therefore may require higher doses and more potent inotropic agents than would be necessary for the left ventricle. Another goal of inotropic agents for patients with right ventricular dysfunction is to increase right ventricular coronary blood flow to improve myocardial performance and therefore cardiac output. The determinants of coronary blood flow are different for the right ventricle compared to the left ventricle.[78] Under the normal low-pressure condition of the right ventricle, the majority of myocardial coronary blood flow occurs during ventricular systole. This is in contrast to the left ventricle, which is a higher pressure system and where the majority of the myocardial blood flow occurs during diastole. Therefore, in patients with right ventricular dysfunction (and normal right ventricular pressures), a normal or elevated systolic pressure can increase myocardial blood flow and augment contractility. The goal of vasoactive agents in patients with right ventricular dysfunction is to increase the force of contractility and increase coronary flow to the right ventricle by increasing systolic pressure. The initial therapy to improve right ventricular output is usually dopamine at 5 to 15 µg/kg. The right

Right   Ventricular   Dysfunction

Diagnosis: Decreased oxygen delivery due to decreased cardiac output

Treatment: Increase cardiac output

1. **Optimize heart rate**
   Improved
   ↓ No

2. **Optimize Preload**
   (RAP< 15 mmHg)
   Improved
   ↓ No

3. **Augment coronary perfusion pressures and RV function**

   Inotropes
   Calcium
   Neosynephrine
   Dopamine
   Epinepherine
   Dobutamine

   Improved
   ↓ No

4. **Reduce Afterload**
   See treatment of Pulmonary hypertension

   Improved
   ↓ No

5. **Evaluate for Anatomic Problems**
   Repair in OR or Interventional Cath Lab

   Improved
   ↓ No

6. **ECMO, RVAD**

FIGURE 1–4.   Decision-making algorithm for postoperative congenital cardiac patients with right ventricular dysfunction. Important concerns are preload augmentation, reducing pulmonary vascular resistance, and maintaining coronary perfusion. ECMO, extracorporeal membrane oxygenation; RVAD, right ventricular assist device.

ventricle may be insensitive to catecholamines, and high levels of dopamine may be necessary to improve oxygen delivery. When the patient is refractory to dopamine, epinephrine at low doses may prove beneficial. Isoproterenol is a β-agonist that results in vasodilatation, tachycardia, and a mild increase in contractility. The increase in contractility and decreased afterload created by isoproterenol may be useful in patients with right ventricular dysfunction and pulmonary hypertension. However, isoproterenol should be used cautiously because the tachycardia and decreased afterload that frequently develop result in increased myocardial oxygen demand, decreased coronary blood flow, and possibly right ventricular ischemia. In patients with right ventricular dysfunction and increased right ventricular afterload, a better pharmacological approach is to utilize amrinone which does not cause the tachycardia associated with isoproterenol use.[82]

Patients with right ventricular dysfunction will benefit by manipulations of cardiorespiratory interactions to optimize right ventricular preload and afterload. The development of a ventilatory strategy for these patients requires an understanding of the effects of cardiorespiratory interaction on right ventricular performance. The preload to the right ventricle is derived from the superior vena cava and inferior vena cava which are outside the thorax. The right ventricular stroke volume, however, is delivered within the thorax and directed toward the afterload of the pulmonary circuit. Therefore, changes in intrathoracic pressure can result in dramatic changes in right ventricular preload and afterload.[86,102] Preload augmentation can be performed by reducing the intrathoracic pressures to a minimal level. Right ventricular afterload can be reduced by hyperoxygenation and hyperventilation, and this will be described in detail in the next section. Since the majority of pulmonary blood flow occurs during expiration, inspiratory times should be short compared to expiratory times. Conventional mechanical ventilation in patients with right ventricular dysfunction should be initiated with a tidal volume of 15 ml/kg, a rate of 15 to 20 beats/minute, FIO_2 equal to 1.0, and a long expiratory time. In addition, low levels of PEEP are maintained so that intrathoracic pressure and pulmonary vascular resistance are reduced.

An alternative approach to increased oxygen delivery in patients with right ventricular dysfunction is for the surgeon to leave (or create) an atrial level right-to-left shunt. Patients with right ventricular dysfunction have decreased oxygen delivery due to decreased cardiac output. The decreased right ventricular cardiac output results in a reduction in left ventricular end-diastolic volume and left ventricular output (ventricular interdependence). Patients with right ventricular dysfunction have elevated right atrial pressures, and atrial level shunt allows blood from the high-pressure right atrium to be shunted to the left atrium. This results in an increase in left ventricular end-diastolic volume and improvement in cardiac output. Since oxygen delivery is a function of cardiac output and oxygen content of the blood, oxygen delivery can be improved by preserving cardiac output. These patients will develop systemic arterial desaturation and decreased oxygen content due to the desaturated right atrial blood that enters the left side of the circulation. Oxygen delivery, however, will be increased because of the increase in cardiac output. As right ventricular function improves, right atrial pressure falls (due to improvement in right ventricular compliance), and this reduces the right-to-left shunt and increases oxygen saturation. The majority of these patients do not require future atrial septal defect closure after repair.

An additional maneuver to compensate for right ventricular dysfunction is to leave the sternum open.[101] If ventricular distention or edema has occurred, opening the chest wall will allow the right ventricle to increase its diastolic volume without resulting in a dramatic increase in diastolic pressure. Furthermore, this maneuver eliminates (or diminishes) the negative effects of ventilation on right ventricle filling and afterload. An increase in right ventricular end-diastolic volume will result in an increase in cardiac output and improvement in oxygen delivery. Ventricular assist devices (VADs) and extracorporeal membrane oxygenation (ECMO) have been used successfully in patients with right ventricular dysfunction.[93,96] The indications for initiating this therapy are the same indicators that are used in patients with left ventricular dysfunction. ECMO has been demonstrated to be more effective in patients with right ventricular dysfunction than in patients with left ventricular dysfunction and therefore should be considered when other alternatives are unsuccessful.[93,96]

Pulmonary Hypertension

Pulmonary hypertension is a frequent postoperative condition, especially in neonatal patients. All neonates are at high risk for the development of pulmonary hypertension due to the high pulmonary pressure in utero and increased muscularization of pulmonary arterioles as previously discussed.[103] In addition, infants with increased pulmonary blood flow lesions are at risk for pulmonary hypertensive crisis in the postoperative period. Pulmonary hypertensive crisis remains a significant problem and is the most frequent indication for the use of ECMO.[96] Patients with pulmonary hypertension develop right ventricular dysfunction due to an increase in afterload of the right ventricle.[9] These patients present with clinical signs similar to patients with right ventricular dysfunction. Episodes of acute deterioration, called pulmonary hypertensive crises, can occur and are associated with an acute reduction in oxygen delivery. The overall result of a pulmonary hypertensive crisis is a reduction in cardiac output from the right ventricle because it is unable to respond to the increased afterload. When a pulmonary hypertensive crisis occurs, the episode is severe and leads to metabolical acidosis with a further reduction of right ventricular cardiac output. A cyclical crisis can develop where increasing acidosis results in increased pulmonary vascular resistance and pulmonary artery pressure, further decreasing cardiac output which then results in further acidosis. The diagnosis of pulmonary hypertension requires demonstration of increased pulmonary artery pressures, increased right heart pressures, right ventricular dysfunction, decreased cardiac output, and decreased oxygen delivery. Decreased oxygen delivery will be manifest by cool extremities, decreased capillary refill, systemic arterial desaturation, and increased heart rate.

Therapy for pulmonary artery hypertension is directed at immediately lowering pulmonary artery pressures and improving right ventricular function by optimizing preload and contractility (Fig. 1–2).[9,10,14,103] Patients with elevated pulmonary vascular resistance are sensitive to changes in right ventricular preload. Because of the increased afterload, the right ventricle will require increased right ventricular preload in order to maximize right ventricular stroke volume. Therefore, these patients require an assessment of right-sided filling pressures and higher than usual filling pressures (right atrial pressure, 10 to 12 mm Hg). As afterload increases, the end-systolic volume of the right ventricle increases. An increase in right ventricular end-diastolic and end-systolic volume can result in conformational changes in the intraventricular septum which can cause a reduction of left ventricular volume and a reduction of left ventricular stroke volume.[104] Because of the decreased right ventricular cardiac output demonstrated in the majority of these patients, inotropic agents are frequently utilized. However, there has been very limited success in using inotropic agents in patients with pulmonary artery hypertension. This may be related to the relative insensitivity of the right ventricle to inotropes. Furthermore, this approach does not treat the increased right ventricular afterload which is the primary pathophysiological disturbance. Agents such as dopamine, epinephrine, and dobutamine have limited utility in treating patients with pulmonary hypertensive crisis, and these patients are more successfully treated by decreasing the right ventricular afterload.

Attempts to manipulate pulmonary vascular resistance through pharmacological intervention have been unsatisfactory. Pharmacological agents that have shown the greatest promise in reducing right ventricular afterload have been the phosphodiesterase inhibitors.[80,82] Amrinone is the only drug in this class commonly available in this country that has been shown to cause a reduction in pulmonary vascular resistance, systemic vascular resistance, and an increase in cardiac output in selected patients. Another nonselective pulmonary vasodilator is isoproterenol, which is a β_1- and β_2-agonist that has mild pulmonary artery vasodilating properties in the normal pulmonary circulation.[105,106] Isoproterenol has been shown to reduce pulmonary vascular resistance in adults after cardiac transplant. Immature animals have been shown to be less responsive to isoproterenol compared to older animals, and this may be true in neonatal patients as well.[105] As discussed previously, isoproterenol can produce tachycardia and myocardial ischemia, which may be especially problematic in patients with right ventricular hypertension due to an increased afterload, which already has a high oxygen need. We, therefore, recommend cautious use of isoproterenol in patients with increased pulmonary artery pressures in the postoperative period. Two other agents used to reduce right ventricular afterload are prostaglandin E_1 and prostacyclin (PGI_2).[14,15] These agents have been shown to promote a reduction in pulmonary artery pressures, but neither of these drugs are selective pulmonary vasodilators, and systemic vasodilatation also occurs. Their use is often limited by systemic hypotension, which can be severe and require another inotrope such as norepinephrine infused directly into the left circulation via a LA line. Because of the vasodilating property, both agents can reduce preload and may result in a reduction in stroke volume due to a reduction in end-diastolic volume. Therefore, careful attention to the intravascular volume status is required, and these patients may require volume expanders during the initiation of prostaglandin therapy. PGI_2 infusions have successfully been used in Europe to prevent a pulmonary hypertensive crisis in patients after surgery for congenital heart disease.[107]

Pharmacological manipulation of the pulmonary vasculature tone is limited by the nonselectivity of the agents available, and because of this lack of specificity, newer pharmacological methods of manipulating the pulmonary vasculature are being sought. Two new concepts include ultrashort acting intravenous vasodilators and inhaled vasoactive agents. Ultrashort acting vasodilators are nonselective vasodilators with a half-life measured in seconds. Infusion of these drugs into the right heart produces a potent short-lived relaxation in the pulmonary artery smooth muscle, and when the drug reaches the systemic circulation, it is no longer active. These drugs, which include adenosine and adenosine triphosphate-like compounds, may have clinical applicability in pulmonary hypertension.[108]

Nitric oxide (NO) has been shown to be effective in treating pulmonary artery hypertension in patients with congenital heart disease. NO is a reactive byproduct of combustion and considered an important toxic gas responsible for a portion of morbidity associated with air pollution.[109,110] Recent studies have identified NO as an important endogenous biological mediator of vascular tone, platelet function, neurotransmission, inflammation, and immune responses. Nitric oxide is produced in endothelial cells by conversion of L-arginine to L-citrulline and NO. The reaction is regulated by the enzyme nitric oxide synthase (NOS) located within the endothelial cells.[111] NO freely diffuses to the surrounding tissues including subjacent vascular smooth muscle where it activates the soluble form of guanylate cyclase and increases cyclic guanosine 3', 5'-monophosphate (cGMP) causing smooth muscle relaxation.[112,113] Any NO that diffuses into the vascular space binds with a high affinity to hemoglobin (about 3000 times that of oxygen),[114] forming nitrosylhemoglobin and thereby becoming inactivated. In the presence of oxygen nitrosylhemoglobin is oxidized to methemoglobin and metabolized to nitrites and nitrates which are then excreted in the urine.[115-117] Therefore, the high affinity of nitric oxide to hemoglobin and the rapid inactivation limit inhaled nitric oxide's activity to the pulmonary vascular bed, resulting in selective pulmonary vasodilation.

Nitric oxide, or endothelial-derived relaxing factor, can be administered as an inhaled gas. It is a nonselective vasodilator which is rapidly inactivated by hemoglobin.[118] When inhaled, nitric oxide results in rapid vasodilatation of pulmonary arteries and reduction in pulmonary vascular resistance. Inhaled nitric oxide has virtually no effect on the systemic circulation because it is rapidly inactivated by hemoglobin. A prompt reduction in pulmonary vascular resistance has been demonstrated after the inhalation of nitric oxide in several clinical settings, including that of newborns with pulmonary artery hypertension.[119] Newborns with pulmonary artery hypertension either alone or in association with meconium aspiration have a high mortality owing to decreased oxygen delivery from right-to-left intracardiac or ductal shunting secondary to pulmonary artery hypertension. In an animal model of neonatal hypertension, Frostell demonstrated that nitric oxide blunted hypoxic pulmonary vasoconstriction, which lowered pulmonary artery pressure, reduced the right-to-left shunting, and improved oxygen delivery.[117] The success of this laboratory experiment has stimulated several clinical studies which have demonstrated that in selected patients nitric oxide results in a lowering of pulmonary artery pressure and improved oxygen saturations.[118,120] Why some patients respond better than others is not understood, but this question may be answered in the ongoing randomized clinical trials. In addition, the best mode of ventilation and the best method of delivering nitric oxide are also in question. The role of nitric oxide in newborns with pulmonary artery hypertension has already decreased the number of infants that require extracorporeal membrane oxygenation in many centers.

Nitric oxide has been used successfully in patients with pulmonary artery hypertension after surgery for congenital heart disease.[121] Patients who are at high risk for the development of pulmonary artery hypertensive crisis in the postoperative period include patients with large left-to-right shunts in the preoperative period. When a pulmonary artery hypertensive crisis develops in these patients a critical decrease in oxygen delivery can occur having a crescendo course. Many of these patients will have a decrease in pulmonary artery pressure and more favorable postoperative hemodynamics after the initiation of nitric oxide.[122] In these patients nitric oxide may be initiated prophylactically in the perioperative period in high-risk patients.

Another pharmacological approach used to alleviate pulmonary artery hypertension is the use of potent opioids to extend the anesthetic period through the first 24 to 48 hours postoperatively.[123–125] Narcotic-based analgesic regimens have been shown to prevent systemic-mediated increases in pulmonary vascular resistance. A continuous infusion of fentanyl or fentanyl plus midazolam may be particularly useful in patients who develop labile pulmonary artery hypertension or hypertensive crises. In a study of newborns after cardiac surgery, administration of fentanyl prior to endotracheal suctioning prevented the development of reactive pulmonary artery hypertension.[116] The effects of fentanyl are most likely due to an attenuated release of the endogenous sympathetic mediators, such as epinephrine and norepinephrine, that produce a vasoconstrictor effect on pulmonary artery smooth muscle. The use of continuous infusion of opioids, such as fentanyl or sufentanyl alone or in combination with a benzodiazepine (midazolam), is now considered to be routine postoperative care for patients with pulmonary artery hypertension.[125,126] Neuromuscular blocking agents should be considered in all patients with agitation or increased sensitivity to small changes in the pattern of ventilation or changes in $PaCO_2$. Neuromuscular blockade allows for a more precise control of ventilation, pH, and $PaCO_2$, thus optimizing therapy based on improving pulmonary vascular resistance.

One of the most successful approaches to reduce pulmonary artery pressures is the manipulation of cardiorespiratory interactions to lower pulmonary vascular resistance. Therapy directed at reducing pulmonary hypertension consists of increasing pH, decreasing $PaCO_2$, increasing PaO_2 and PAO_2, and minimizing intrathoracic pressures.[9,10,86,127–129] Increasing pH has been shown to significantly reduce pulmonary vascular resistance in a variety of studies. Drummond et al. showed that by reducing $Paco_2$ to 20 and increasing pH to 7.6, a consistent reduction of pulmonary vascular resistance is obtained in infants with pulmonary hypertension. In addition, maintaining serum bicarbonate levels at a pH between 7.5 to 7.6 while maintaining a $Paco_2$ of 40 resulted in a similar reduction in pulmonary vascular resistance.[8,119,120] Both an increase in pH and a reduction in $Paco_2$ could independently result in a reduction in right ventricular afterload. Other studies have shown that an increase in both alveolar oxygen (Pao_2) and arterial oxygen (Pao_2) by increasing inspired oxygen concentration can also result in a reduction of pulmonary vascular resistance.[10,11] Increasing inspired oxygen increased Pao_2 in patients without a shunt and resulted in a reduction of pulmonary artery vascular resistance. Increasing inspired oxygen in patients with intracardiac shunts resulted in little change in Pao_2; however, a reduction in pulmonary vascular resistance occurred. This was related to an increase in Pao_2 and demonstrates that an increase in both alveolar and arterial oxygen content can alter pulmonary vascular resistance. In animal studies, increasing inspired oxygen concentration has been shown to be a more potent pulmonary vasodilator in neonates than in the adult.[11] The use of inspired oxygen to reduce pulmonary vascular resistance has been useful in the ICU and is a frequent mode of interrogating pulmonary vascular responsiveness in the cardiac catheterization laboratory.[11]

Mechanical ventilation is usually required in patients with pulmonary artery hypertension. The effects of different types of ventilation on pulmonary vascular resistance are not well established. A reduction in mean airway pressure will reduce pulmonary vascular resistance.[86] Patients with pulmonary artery hypertension may benefit from hyperventilation, but because of the detrimental effects of mean airway pressure on pulmonary vascular resistance and right ventricular filling, mean airway pressure should be limited.[9] Therefore, PEEP must be used judiciously in these patients. Low PEEP (2 to 3 mm Hg) may be helpful in preventing collapse of the alveoli, but high PEEP or high mean airway pressure will result in alveolar overdistention and compression of the pulmonary capillaries with a resultant increase in pulmonary vascular resistance.[12] Therefore, an approach to these patients based on the pathophysiology of pulmonary artery hypertension should be directed at reducing right ventricular afterload and improving the right ventricular stroke volume by increasing right ventricular preload.

Several differences in lung physiology exist in newborns and infants compared to adults.[83,85,88,129] At the end of normal breathing many of the smaller infants have reduced functional residual capacity and increased airway collapse. This process results in a ventilation-perfusion mismatch with segments of lung demonstrating perfusion without ventilation.[130,131] As these nonventilated lung segments become hypoxic, a secondary hypoxic response can develop, and pulmonary vascular resistance elevates.[8] In order to increase lung volumes at the end of inspiration without increasing mean airway pressure, large tidal volumes of 15 to 20 ml/kg are required. Respiratory rates are usually held at 15 to 20 beats/minute, and respiratory cycles with short inspiratory times and long expiratory phases are utilized to augment pulmonary blood flow. The short inspiratory time and low rates help to minimize mean airway pressure. In addition, PEEP is held at the minimum required to prevent atelectasis.

Because of the detrimental effects of positive pressure ventilation on right ventricular dynamics and the need for hyperventilation, alternate modes of ventilation have been tried for patients with pulmonary hypertension and right ventricular dysfunction. High-frequency jet ventilation (HFJV) is an alternative mode of ventilation for these patients.[86] Because HFJV reduces mean airway pressure and pulmonary vascular resistance while maintaining a similar $PaCO_2$, it should be ideally suited for patients with right ventricular dysfunction and/or pulmonary artery hypertension. In postoperative Fontan patients whose cardiac index is dramatically dependent on mean airway pressure and pulmonary vascular resistance, HFJV decreases mean airway pressure 50%, reduces pulmonary vascular resistance by 64%, and increases the cardiac index by 24% (Fig. 1–3).[86]

ECMO, which has been used effectively in neonatal patients with pulmonary hypertension, may also be beneficial for selected patients with pulmonary hypertension in the postoperative period.[93,96]

Presence of Residual Lesions

The presence of residual structural defects can result in abnormal convalescence and should be vigorously investigated whenever there is an unexplained postoperative course or complications refractory to routine maneuvers. A clear understanding of the anatomy and physiology of the repair is necessary in order to appropriately assess for hemodynamically significant residual lesions. The presence of residual lesions can be categorized into four groups: 1) residual shunts; 2) residual stenosis/insufficiency; 3) residual anatomical defects related to the underlying defect; and 4) arrhythmias. All significant residual lesions result in a reduction of oxygen delivery or an abnormal oxygen supply to demand ratio of the myocardium. Although arrhythmias may not always truly be a residual defect, they can be a result of surgery or develop after surgical intervention and, therefore, can be classified as a residual problem resulting in decreased oxygen delivery and abnormal convalescence. The diagnosis of residual lesions is performed by intraoperative evaluation or postoperative echocardiography and cardiac catheterization. Patients may have evidence of residual disease by physical examination or through a pattern of abnormal postoperative convalescence. Physical exam can provide information about shunts and valvular function by demonstrating the presence of new or abnormal murmurs. In addition, decreased oxygen delivery can also be demonstrated. Noninvasive testing including pulse oximetry and chest x-rays may be helpful in demonstrating the presence of significant residual lesions. Patients with persistent metabolical acidosis or elevated lactate levels despite medical intervention should be aggressively evaluated for the presence of residual cardiac lesions.

Echocardiography and cardiac catheterization should be directed at evaluating the integrity of the repair. The type, extent, and tolerance of residual cardiac defects are dependent upon the method of repair. In patients who have undergone complete reconstruction, residual defects occur at areas of anastamoses or intracardiac shunt closure. In patients who require physiological reconstruction, e.g., palliation, residual anatomical defects may be less tolerated due to the abnormal loading conditions that exist in the preoperative period and because of an abnormal pattern of flow after surgery. Patients who have a residual intracardiac shunt should have aggressive evaluation of the hemodynamic significance of the shunt. A residual shunt can usually be documented by echocardiography and assessed by cardiac catheterization. A residual intracardiac left-to-right shunt of $>2.0/1.0$ is poorly tolerated and usually indicates the need for intervention. Small shunts may be hemodynamically insignificant in individual patients and should be cautiously interpreted along with other indicators of abnormal convalescence. The presence of a residual stenosis is usually poorly tolerated in the postoperative period, because it results in increased afterload to the ventricle, decreased oxygen delivery, and increased oxygen consumption. The need for intervention in patients with a residual stenosis must be individualized. If decreased oxygen delivery is refractory to medical management, any residual stenosis should be removed. As an example, a small residual aortic arch gradient in a patient after stage I reconstruction for hypoplastic left heart syndrome is usually associated with significantly reduced oxygen delivery and is poorly tolerated. This should be compared to patients after surgery for tetralogy of Fallot who demonstrate a residual outflow tract gradient which is usually well tolerated. Valvar insufficiency results in increased preload to the ventricle and volume overloading.

This is usually better tolerated in the postoperative period than valvular stenosis inasmuch as cardiac output can usually be maintained through ventricular dilation with an increase in end-diastolic volume. Significant insufficiency, however, can lead to a reduction in oxygen delivery as a result of decreased cardiac output. Echocardiography and cardiac catheterization play a pivotal role in determining the hemodynamic significance of valvular insufficiency. The need to intervene is individualized and based on persistence of decreased oxygen delivery due to valvar insufficiency.

Some residual defects are irreparable and reflect underlying anatomical deficiencies inherent in the congenital heart defect. For example, some patients with aortic coarctation or critical aortic stenosis have associated left ventricular chamber hypoplasia. It is generally considered that a left ventricular volume less than 20 ml/m² is incompatible with acceptable function. Patients who have left ventricular volumes approximating this value may present with variable degrees of heart failure following coarctation repair (or aortic valvotomy). This "residual" anatomical problem is a feature of the underlying defect. In some cases, leaving the ductus arteriosus open on PGE₁ has been reported in these patients to decompress the pulmonary circuit until the LV compliance improves.[132] Likewise, the presence of endocardial fibroelastosis, mitral valve hypoplasia, or a restrictive aortic annulus may complicate the recovery of infants following aortic valvotomy for critical aortic stenosis. In some cases, these "residual defects" may prove lethal, despite excellent postoperative care. Therefore, the intensive care physician must appreciate that the nature of many congenital heart lesions is complex and not always compatible with normal or even successful convalescence.

Arrhythmias can occur in the postoperative setting and require treatment. Most patients undergoing repair of congenital heart lesions have temporary atrial and ventricular pacing wires placed in the operating room, and these can be especially helpful in diagnosing and treating postoperative arrhythmias.[133] Arrhythmias can occur as a result of the surgical procedure, e.g., complete heart block following VSD closure; as a result of the defect, e.g., atrial arrhythmias following atrial switch for transposition and ventricular dysrhythmias from the cardiomyopathy associated with anomalous coronary arteries; as a result of cardioplegia, e.g., transient supraventricular dysrhythmias; or as a result of the postoperative therapy, e.g., various tachycardias induced by inotropic agents. Regardless of the cause of arrhythmias, they can present problems which must be dealt with effectively by the intensive care staff, and they can be a significant reason for postoperative morbidity and mortality.

SUMMARY

The perioperative approach requires a coordinated, multidisciplinary approach to patient care and, as such, requires input from pediatric cardiologists, pediatric cardiac surgeons, pediatric intensivists, pediatric cardiovascular anesthesiologists, perfusionists, specialized nurses, and respiratory therapists. Treatment is directed at optimizing oxygen delivery and minimizing the toxicities associated with the therapies utilized. By utilizing the principles outlined above, a multidisciplinary approach can be achieved and patient care optimized.

References

1. Groh MA, et al: Repair of tetralogy of Fallot in infancy: Effect of pulmonary artery size on outcome. Circulation 84:III206–III212, 1991
2. Lupinetti FM, et al: Intermediate-term survival and functional results after arterial repair for transposition of the great arteries. J Thorac Cardiovasc Surg 103:421–427, 1992
3. Castaneda AR, et al: The neonate with critical congenital heart disease: Repair—a surgical challenge. J Thorac Cardiovasc Surg, 98(5(part 2)):869, 1989
4. Shoemaker WC, et al: Hemodynamic and oxygen transport monitoring to titrate therapy in septic shock. New Horizons 1(1):145–159, 1993
5. Lister G, et al: Effects of alterations of oxygen transport on the neonate. Semin Perinatol 8(3):192–204, 1984
6. Guyton AC: Textbook of Medical Physiology. Philadelphia, WB Saunders, 1981
7. Meliones JN, et al: Longitudinal results following the first stage palliation for hypoplastic left heart syndrome. Circulation 82((suppl IV)): IV151–IV156, 1990
8. Rudolph AM, Yuan S: Response of the pulmonary vasculature to hypoxia and H+ ion concentration changes. J Clin Invest 45:399, 1966
9. Drummond WH, et al: The independent effects of hyperventilation, tolazoline, and dopamine in infants with persistent pulmonary hypertension. J Pediatr 98:603–608, 1981
10. Custer JR, Hales CA: Influence of alveolar oxygen on pulmonary vasoconstriction in newborn lambs vs sheep. Am Rev Respir Dis 132:326, 1985
11. Lock JE, Einjig S, Bass JL: Pulmonary vascular response to oxygen and its influence on operative results in children with ventricular septal defects. Pediatr Cardiol 3:41, 1982
12. Hammon JW, et al: The effect of positive end expiratory pressure on regional ventilation and perfusion in the normal and injured primate lung. J Thorac Cardiovasc Surg 72:680, 1976
13. McGoon DC, Mair DD: On the unmuddling of shunting, mixing and streaming. J Thorac Cardiovasc Surg 100(1):77, 1990
14. Drummond WH, Lock JE: Neonatal pulmonary vasodilator drugs. Dev Pharmacol Ther 7:1, 1984
15. Heymann MA, Hoffman JIE: Persistent pulmonary hypertension syndromes in the newborn. In Weir EK, Reeves JT (eds): Pulmonary Hypertension. New York, Futura, 1984

16. Norwood WI, M. JD: Hypoplastic left heart syndrome. In Sabiston DC, Spencer FC (Eds): Surgery of the Chest, pp. 1493–1502. Philadelphia, WB Saunders, 1990

17. Nicolson SC, Jobes DR: Hypoplastic left heart syndrome. In Lake CL (ed): Pediatric Cardiac Anesthesia, pp. 243–252. Norwalk, Appleton & Lange, 1988

18. Hansen DD, Hickey PR: Anesthesia for hypoplastic left heart syndrome: Use of high-dose fentanyl in 30 neonates. Anesth Analg 65:127–132, 1986

19. Ungerleider RM, et al: Routine use of intraoperative epicardial echo and Doppler color flow imaging to guide and evaluate repair of congenital heart lesions: A prospective study. J Thorac Cardiovasc Surg 100(2):297, 1990

20. Ungerleider RM, et al: The learning curve for intraoperative echocardiography during congenital heart surgery. Ann Thorac Surg 54:691–698, 1992

21. Hsu YH, et al. Impact of intraoperative echocardiography on surgical management of congenital heart disease. Am J Cardiol 67:1279–1283, 1991

22. Dan M, et al: Value of transesophageal echocardiography during repair of congenital heart defects. Ann Thorac Surg 50:637–643, 1990

23. Sutherland GR, et al: Epicardial and transesophageal echocardiography during surgery for congenital heart disease. Int J Card Imaging 4:37–40, 1989

24. Ungerleider RM: The use of intraoperative epicardial echocardiography with color flow imaging during the repair of complete atrioventricular septal defects. Cardiol Young 2:56–64, 1992

25. Ungerleider RM, et al: The use of intraoperative echo with Doppler color flow imaging to predict outcome after repair of congenital heart defects. Ann Surg 210(4):526–534, 1989

26. Ungerleider RM: Epicardial echocardiography during repair of congenital heart defects. In Advances in Cardiac Surgery. St. Louis, Mosby-Year Book, 1992

27. Moorthy SS, et al: Transient right-left shunt during emergence from anesthesia demonstrated by color flow Doppler mapping. Anesth Analg 68: 20–22, 1989

28. Moorthy SS, et al: Transient hypoxemia from a transient right to left shunt in a child during emergence from anesthesia. Anesthesiology 66: 234–235, 1987

29. Nundel D, Berman N, Talner N: Effects of acutely increasing systemic vascular resistance on arterial oxygen tension in tetralogy of Fallot. Pediatrics 58:248–251, 1976

30. Parr GVS, Blackstone EH, Kirklin JW: Cardiac performance and mortality early after intracardiac surgery in infants and young children. Circulation 51:867–871, 1975

31. Gold JP, et al: Transthoracic intracardiac monitoring lines in pediatric surgical patients: A ten year experience. Ann Thorac Surg 42:185, 1986

32. Lang P, Chipman CW, Siden H: Early assessment of hemodynamic states after repair of tetralogy of Fallot: A comparison of 24 hour (intensive care unit) and 1 year postoperative data in 98 patients. Am J Cardiol 50: 795–801, 1982

33. Jenkins J, et al: Effects of mechanical ventilation on cardiopulmonary function in children after open-heart surgery. Crit Care Med 13:77–80, 1985

34. Jarmakani JM, et al: Effect of extracellular calcium on myocardial mechanical function in neonatal rabbit. Dev Pharmacol Ther 5:1–13, 1982
35. Rebeyka IM, et al: Altered contractile response in neonatal myocardium to citrate-phophate-dextrose infusion. Circulation 82:IV-367–IV-370, 1990
36. Meliones JN, et al: Hemodynamic instability after the initiation of extracorporeal membrane oxygenation: The role of ionized calcium. Crit Care Med 19:1247, 1991
37. Rosenthal SM, LaJohn LA: Effect of age on transvascular fluid movement. Am J Physiol 228:134–139, 1975
38. Haneda K, Sato S, Ischizawa E: The importance of colloid osmotic pressure during open heart surgery in infants. Tohoku J Exp Med 147:65–71, 1985
39. Minich LA, et al: Echocardiographic assessment following the arterial switch procedure. Dyna Cardiol Imag 1(1):30–40, 1991
40. Meliones JN, et al: Doppler evaluation of homograft vs. left ventriculated conduits in children. Am J Cardiol 64:354–358, 1989
41. Meliones JN, et al: Pulsed Doppler assessment of left ventricular diastolic filling in children with left ventricular outflow obstruction before and after balloon angioplasty. Am J Cardiol 63:231–236, 1989
42. Meliones JN, Snider AR, B. EL, Echocardiographic assessment following the Norwood procedure. Dyna Cardiovasc Imag 2(4):225–234, 1989
43. Frommelt PC, et al: Doppler assessment of pulmonary artery flow patterns and ventricular function after the Fontan operation. Am J Cardiol 68:1211–1215, 1991
44. Ungerleider RM, et al: Routine use of intraoperative epicardial echocardiography and Doppler color flow imaging to guide and evaluate repair of congenital heart defects. J Thorac Cardiovasc Surg 100:297–309, 1990
45. Mullins CE: Pediatric and congenital therapeutic cardiac catheterization. Circulation 79:1153–1159, 1989
46. Berner M, Rouge JC, Friedli B: The hemodynamic effect of phentolamine and dobutamine after open-heart operations in children: Influence of underlying heart defect. Ann Thorac Surg 35:643–650, 1983
47. Borow KM, et al: Left ventricular function after repair of tetralogy of Fallot and its relationship to age at surgery. Circulation, 61:1150, 1980
48. Borow KM, et al: Systemic ventricular function in patients with tetralogy of Fallot ventricular septal defect and transposition of the great arteries repaired during infancy. Circulation 64:878, 1981
49. Graham TP, et al: Left ventricular wall stress and contractile function in childhood: Normal values and comparison of Fontan repair versus palliation only in patients with tricuspid atresia. Circulation 74(suppl): 61–69, 1986
50. Baylen B, Meyer RA, Korfhagen J: Left ventricular performance in the critically ill premature infant with patent ductus arteriosus and pulmonary disease. Circulation 55:182–188, 1977
51. Jarmakani JM, Graham TP, Canent RV: Left ventricular contractile state in children with successfully corrected ventricular septal defect. Circulation suppl I(I102–I110), 1972
52. Nishioka K, et al: Left ventricular volume characteristics in children with tricuspid atresia before and after surgery. Am J Cardiol 47:1105–1107, 1981
53. Nasser R, Reedy MC, Anderson PAW: Developmental changes in the ultrastructure and sarcomere shortening of the isolated rabbit myocardium. Circ Res 61:465, 1987

54. Humpherys JE, Cummings P: Atrial and ventricular tropomysin and tro-ponin-I in the developing bovine and human heart. J Mol Cell Cardiol 16:643, 1984

55. Legato MJ: Ultrastructural changes during normal growth in the dog and rat ventricular myofiber. In Developmental and Physiological Correlates of Cardiac Muscle, p. 249. S.T. Lieberman M, Editor. New York, Raven Press, 1975

56. Vetter R, et al: Developmental changes of Ca++ transport systems in chick heart. Biomed Biochim Acta 45(S219), 1986

57. Driscoll DJ, et al: Comparative hemodynamic effects of isoproterenol, dopamine and dobutamine in the newborn dog. Pediatr Res 13:1006, 1979

58. Friedman WF: The intrinsic physiologic properties of the developing heart. Prog Cardiovasc Dis 15:87, 1972

59. Becker AE, Caruso G: Congenital heart disease—a morphologist's view on myocardial dysfunction. In Becker AE, Marcelleti C, Anderson RH (eds): Paediatric Cardiology. Edinburgh, Churchill Livingstone, 1981

60. Romero TE, F. WF: Limited left ventricular response to volume overload in the neonatal period: A comparative study with the adult animal. Pediatr Res 13:910, 1979

61. Thornburg KL, Morton MJ: Filling and arterial pressure as determinants of RV stroke volume in the sheep fetus. Am J Physiol 244:H656–H663, 1983

62. Kirkpatrick SE, Johnson GH, Assali NS: Frank-Starling as an important determinant of fetal cardiac output. Am J Physiol 231:495–500, 1976

63. Teitel DF, et al: Developmental changes in myocardial contractile reserve in the lamb. Pediatr Res 19:948–955, 1985

64. Cheng JB, et al: Identification of beta-adrenergic receptors using [H]dihydroalprenolol in fetal sheep heart: Direct evidence of qualitative similarity to the receptors in adult sheep heart. Pediatr Res 15:1083,

65. Vapaavouri EK, et al: Development of cardiovascular response to auto-nomic blockade in intact fetal and neonatal lambs. Biol Neonate 22:177, 1973

66. Gootman N, et al: Maturation-related differences in regional circulatory effects of dopamine infusion in swine. Dev Pharmacol Ther 6:9, 1983

67. Buckley NM, Brazeau P, F. ID: Cardiovascular effects of dopamine in developing swine. Biol Neonate 43:50, 1983

68. Seguchi M, Harding JA, J. JM, Developmental change in the function of sarcoplasmic reticulum. J Mol Cell Cardiol 18:189, 1986

69. Stephenson LW, et al: Effects of nitroprusside and dopamine on pulmo-nary artery vasculature in children after cardiac surgery. Circulation 60:(suppl)I-104–I-110, 1979

70. Goldberg LI: Cardiovascular and renal actions of dopamine: Potential clinical applications. Pharmacol Rev 24:1, 1972

71. Lang P, Williams RG, Norwood WI: The hemodynamic effects of dopa-mine in infants after corrective cardiac surgery. J Pediatr 96:630, 1980

72. Driscoll DJ, Gillette PC, Fukushige J: Comparison of the cardiovascular action of isoproterenol, dopamine and dobutamine in the neonatal and mature dog. Pediatr Cardiol 1:307, 1980

73. Nakanishi T, Seguchi M, Takao A: Intracellular calcium concentrations in the newborn myocardium. Circulation 76:(suppl)IV-455–IV-461, 1987

74. Bohn DJ, Piorier CS, Edmonds JF: Hemodynamic effects of dobutamine after cardiopulmonary bypass in children. Crit Care Med 8:367–342, 1980

75. Bohn DJ, Poirer CS, Edmonds JF, et al: Efficacy of dopamine, dobutamine, and epinephrine during emergence from cardiopulmonary bypass in children. Crit Care Med 8:367–372, 1980
76. Hess W, Arnold B, Veit S: The hemodynamic effects of amrinone in patients with mitral stenosis and pulmonary hypertension. Eur Heart J 7: 800–807, 1986
77. Lawless S, Burckart G, Diven W: Amrinone pharmacokinetics in neonates and infants. J Clin Pharmacol 28:283, 1988
78. Berne RM, Levy MN: Coronary circulation and cardiac metabolism. In Berne RM, Levy MN (eds): Cardiovascular Physiology. St. Louis, CV Mosby, 1981
79. Park IS, Michael LH, Driscoll DJ: Comparative responses of the developing canine myocardium to inotropic agents. Am J Physiol 242:H13, 1982
80. Konstam MA, Cohen SR, Salem DN: Effect of amrinone on right ventricular function: Predominance of afterload reduction. Circulation 74: 359–366, 1986
81. Konstam MA, Cohen SR, Weiland DS, et al: Relative contribution of inotropic and vasodilator effects to amrinone-induced hemodynamic improvement in congestive heart failure. Am J Cardiol 57:242–248, 1986
82. Wessel DL, Triedman JK, Wernovsky G: Pulmonary and systemic hemodynamics of amrinone in neonates following cardiopulmonary bypass. Circulation 80(suppl II):II488, 1989
83. Fagan DG: Shape changes in V-P loops for children's lungs related to growth. Thorax 32:198, 1977
84. Deal CW, Warden JC, Monk I: Effect of hypothermia on lung compliance. Thorax 25:105–109, 1970
85. Nelson NM: Neonatal pulmonary function. Pediatr Clin North Am 13: 769, 1966
86. Meliones JN, et al: High-frequency jet ventilation improves cardiac function after the Fontan procedure. Circulation 84(suppl III):III-364–III-368, 1991
87. Robotham JL, et al: The effects of positive end-respiratory pressure on right and left ventricular performance. Am Rev Respir Dis 121:677, 1980
88. Zapletal A, Paul T, Samenek M: Pulmonary elasticity in children and adolescents. J Appl Physiol 40:953, 1976
89. Weisfeldt ML, H. HL: Cardiopulmonary resuscitation: Beyond cardiac massage. Circulation 74:443–448, 1986
90. Veasy GL, et al: Intra-aortic balloon pumping in infants and children. Circulation 68(5):1095–1100, 1983
91. Veasy GL, W. H: Intra-aortic balloon pumping in children. Heart Lung 14(6):548–555, 1985
92. del Nido PJ, et al: Successful use of intraaortic balloon pumping in a 2-kilogram infant. Ann Thorac Surg 46:574–576, 1988
93. Meliones JN, et al: Extracorporeal life support for cardiac assist in pediatric patients. Circulation 84(suppl III):III-168–III-172, 1991
94. Pollock JC, et al: Intraaortic balloon pumping in children. Ann Thorac Surg 29(6):522–528, 1980
95. Karl TR, et al: Centrifugal pump left heart assist in pediatric cardiac operations. J Thorac Cardiovasc Surg 102:624–630, 1991
96. Berner M, et al: Chronotropic and inotropic supports are both required to increase cardiac output early after corrective operations for tetralogy of Fallot. J Thorac Cardiovasc Surg 97:297–302, 1989

97. Hines R, Barash PG: Right ventricular failure. In Kaplan JA (ed): Cardiac Anesthesia, 2nd ed., vol. 2. New York, Grune & Stratton, 1987

98. Hilberman M, Myers BD, Carrie et al: Acute renal failure following cardiac surgery. J Thorac Cardiovasc Surg 77:880–888, 1979

99. Perloff J: Development and regression of increased ventricular mass. Am J Cardiol 50:605, 1982

100. Bove AA, S. WP: Ventricular interdependence. Prog Cardiovasc Dis 23: 365, 1981

101. Pearl JM, et al: Repair of truncus arteriosus in infancy. Ann Thorac Surg 52:780–786, 1991

102. Pinsky MR: Determinants of pulmonary arterial flow variation during respiration. J Appl Physiol 56:1237, 1984

103. Rudolph AM: Distribution and regulation of blood flow in the fetal and newborn lamb. Circ Res 57:811, 1985

104. Meyer RA, et al: Ventricular septum in right ventricular volume overload. Am J Cardiol 30:349–354, 1972

105. Molloy DW: Effects of noradrenaline and isoproterenol on cardiopulmonary function in a canine model of acute pulmonary hypertension. Chest 88:432, 1985

106. Schwartz DA, Grove FL, Horowitz LD: Effect of isoproterenol on regional myocardial perfusion and tissue oxygenation in acute myocardial infarction. Am Heart J 97:339, 1979

107. Bush A, Busset C, Knight WB: Modification of pulmonary hypertension secondary to congenital heart disease. Am Rev Respir Dis 136:767, 1987

108. Zall S, Milocco I, Rickstein S-E: Effects of adenosine on myocardial blood flow and metabolism after coronary artery bypass surgery. Anesth Analg 73:689–695, 1991

109. Feldman PL, Griffith OW, Stuehr DJ: The surprising life of nitric oxide. C&EN (December 20):26–38, 1993

110. Pearl RG: Inhaled nitric oxide, the past, the present, and the future. Anesthesiology 78(3):413–416, 1993

111. Palmer RMJ, Ashton DS, Moncada S: Vascular endothelial cells synthesize nitric oxide from L-arginine. Nature 333:664–666, 1988

112. Holzmann S: Endothelium-induced relaxation by acetylcholine associated with larger rises in cGMP in coronary arterial strips. J Cyclic Nucl Res 8:409–419, 1982

113. Ignarro LJ, Burke TM, Wood KS, Wolin MS, Kadowitz PJ: Association between cyclic GMP accumulation and acetylcholine elicited relaxation of bovine intrapulmonary artery. J Pharmacol Exp Ther 228:682–690, 1983

114. Moncada S, Higgs A: The L-arginine-nitric oxide pathway. N Engl J Med 329(27):2002–2012, 1993

115. Ignarro LJ: Biologic actions and properties of endothelium-derived nitric oxide formed and released from artery and vein. Circ Res 65:1–21, 1989

116. Roberts JD: Inhaled nitric oxide for treatment of pulmonary artery hypertension in the newborn and infant. Crit Care Med 21(9):S374–S376, 1993

117. Frostell C, Fratacci MD, Wain JC, Jones R, Zapol WM: Inhaled nitric oxide: A selective pulmonary vasodilator reversing hypoxic pulmonary vasoconstriction. Circulation 83:2038–2047, 1991

118. Frostell CG, Blomqvist H, Hedenstierna G, Lundberg J, Zapol WM: Inhaled nitric oxide selectively reverses human hypoxic pulmonary vasoconstriction without causing systemic vasodilation. Anesthesiology 78: 427–435, 1993

119. Roberts JD, Lang P, Bigatello LM, Vlahakes GJ, Zapol WM: Inhaled nitric oxide in congenital heart disease. Circulation 87(2):447–453, 1993
120. Puybassett L, Stewart T, Rouby JJ, et al: Inhaled nitric oxide reverses the increase in pulmonary vascular resistance induced by permissive hypercapnia in patients with acute respiratory distress syndrome. Anesthesiology 80:1254–1257, 1994
121. Kinsella JP, Neish SR, Schaffer E, et al: Low-dose inhalation of nitric oxide in persistent pulmonary hypertension of the newborn. Lancet 338: 1173–1174, 1991
122. Wessel DL, Adaita I, Thompson JE, Hickey PR: Delivery and monitoring of inhaled nitric oxide in patients with pulmonary hypertension. Crit Care Med 22:930–938, 1994
123. Hickey PR, Hansen DD: Fentanyl and sufentanil-oxygen-pancuronium anesthesia for cardiac surgery in infants. Anesth Analg 63:117, 1984
124. Hickey PR, et al: Blunting of the stress responses in the pulmonary circulation of infants by fentanyl. Anesth Analg 64:1137, 1985
125. Anand KJS, Sippell WG, Aynsley-Green A: Randomized trial of fentanyl anesthesia in preterm neonates undergoing surgery: Effects on the stress response. Lancet 1:243, 1987
126. Greeley WJ, K. F: Anesthesia for pediatric cardiac surgery. In Miller RD (ed): Anesthesia, pp. 1693–1736. New York, Churchill Livingstone, 1990
127. Malik AB, Kidd SL: Independent effects of changes in $H+$ and CO_2 concentrations on hypoxic pulmonary vasoconstriction. J Appl Physiol 34: 318–323, 1973
128. Lyrene RK, et al: Alkalosis attenuates hypoxic pulmonary vasoconstriction in neonatal lambs. Pediatr Res 19(12):1268, 1985
129. Mansell A, Bryan AC: Airway closure in children. J Appl Physiol 33:711, 1972
130. West JB, Dollery CT, N. A: Distribution of blood flow in isolated lung: Relation to vascular and alveolar pressures. J Appl Physiol 19:713, 1964
131. West JB: Respiratory Physiology—The Essentials. Baltimore, Williams & Wilkins, 1979
132. Ungerleider RM: Is there a role for prosthetic patch aortoplasty in the repair of aortic coarctation? Ann Thorac Surg 52:601–603, 1991
133. Waldo AL: Modes and methods of recording electrograms. In Waldo AL, MacLean WAH (eds): Diagnosis and Treatment of Cardiac Arrhythmias Following Open Heart Surgery, p. 21. Mt Kisco, NY, Futura Publishing, 1980

Isobel A. Muhiudeen
Michael K. Cahalan
Norman H. Silverman

Intraoperative Transesophageal Echocardiography in Patients with Congenital Heart Disease

2

Pediatric transesophageal echocardiography (TEE) is a rapidly evolving field, inasmuch as pediatric TEE probes have only recently become available but provide diagnostic information comparable to that achieved with epicardial echocardiography, the technique used during congenital heart surgery since the mid-1980s.[1–5] For example,[6,7] comparative studies demonstrated that both TEE and epicardial echocardiography accurately detected the presence or absence of residual shunts and regurgitation as well as other residual defects.[2,3,5,8] However, when compared to epicardial echocardiography, TEE does not interrupt surgery, cause dysrhythmias, hypotension, or potential infections.[5] As a result, TEE has become a standard of care in many centers for intraoperative and early postoperative evaluation of patients undergoing surgery for congenital heart disease.

INTRAOPERATIVE EPICARDIAL ECHOCARDIOGRAPHY

Color Doppler imaging via epicardial echocardiography is routinely performed intraoperatively in a number of centers[1,7,9] and is the procedure of choice to assess repair of congenital heart defects. Recently, a study from Duke University described the utility of epicardial im-

Perioperative Management of the Patient with Congenital Heart Disease, edited by William J. Greeley. Williams & Wilkins, Baltimore © 1996.

aging for the evaluation of patients undergoing surgical repair of tetralogy of Fallot.[10] Overall, of 31 patients in whom residual VSDs were identified and observed over time, 11 (36%) showed improvement and 15 (48%) showed no change. They concluded that if sizeable defects were noticed by epicardial echocardiography after surgery, a repeat period of cardiopulmonary bypass was indicated. This report and others indicate that epicardial echocardiography is still used despite the availability of high-resolution transesophageal probes,[11] but it should be emphasized that this technique requires participation and concentration by the surgeon. For an excellent and extensive review of epicardial imaging, the reader is referred to an earlier chapter in the Society for Cardiovascular Anesthesia Monographs, 1991.[12]

This chapter will focus on the current practice of tranesophageal echocardiography for congenital heart disease and, in particular, will emphasize a relatively new modality, transgastric imaging.

TEE TECHNIQUE

Transducer Insertion

After the induction of general anesthesia and endotracheal intubation, gastric contents are suctioned. The patient's mouth is opened with the head facing forward, jaw thrust forward, and the neck slightly extended. The lubricated probe is maintained in the unlocked position and gently passed through a bite block into the esophagus. If difficulty is encountered in passing the probe through the hypopharynx, a laryngoscope is used to pass the transducer into the esophagus under direct visualization. Once the transducer is positioned behind the heart, the patient's head can be turned to face the echocardiographer who is manipulating the transducer.

Imaging Technique

The pediatric TEE probe can be manipulated in three directions: advanced or withdrawn, anteflexed or retroflexed, and rotated clockwise or counterclockwise relative to the sagittal plane. As general rules of transducer manipulation, anteflexion of the transducer brings structures anterior and toward the base of the heart into view, clockwise rotation allows imaging of rightward structures, and counterclockwise rotation permits viewing of left-sided structures.

We recommend the image orientation and nomenclature guidelines proposed by the American Society of Echocardiography for the standard basal short-axis, four-chamber, long-axis, and transgastric short-axis transesophageal echocardiographic views.[13]

Short-axis views consist of sectional planes oriented in an axial plane, therefore slightly oblique with respect to a true short-axis view of the heart, ranging from the basal to the transgastric level. The most cranial short-axis view is obtained at the base of the heart from which the probe is anteflexed slightly to display both semilunar valves and the proximal pulmonary artery. Advancement of the probe 0.5 to 1.5 cm displays the proximal ascending aorta and the origins of the coronary arteries. Clockwise rotation of the probe in this position shows the left pulmonary veins; counterclockwise rotation shows the right pulmonary veins, superior vena cava, and right atrial appendage. Further advancement of 0.5 to 1.5 cm demonstrates the interatrial septum, tricuspid valve, and inlet region of the right ventricle. The probe is anteflexed in this position to show the right ventricular outflow tract. By advancing the probe into the stomach, the transgastric short-axis views are obtained with multiple cross-sectional views of the left ventricle, mitral valve, papillary muscles, and oblique views of the right ventricle demonstrated by slight probe flexion and/or rotation at this level.

A transesophageal four-chamber view is demonstrated by withdrawing the probe midway between the transgastric and basal short-axis positions. In this view the atrial, atrioventricular, and ventricular septums and atrioventricular valves are demonstrated. The transesophageal echocardiography long-axis view is obtained by anteflexion and counterclockwise rotation of the probe which displays the left ventricular outflow tract, mitral valve, membranous and muscular regions of the ventricular septum, and an oblique view of the right ventricle.[14] In the smallest patient's (3 to 4 kg), very small adjustments in probe position, i.e., movements of only a few millimeters are required to change from view to view. The distance between the different views increases as the patients weight increases (Fig. 2–1).

Once the standard transverse transesophageal examination is completed, a longitudinal examination can be performed which has been well described elsewhere.[15] However, when only a single-plane probe is available, a complete examination can still be achieved by use of deep transgastric imaging planes: the probe is passed into the stomach, anteflexed maximally, and advanced anteriorly to the fundus. When the patient's abdomen is exposed, it is frequently possible to see the tip of the probe slightly distending the abdominal wall during this maneuver. If there is difficulty in achieving the views the probe is then withdrawn, readvanced, and withdrawn with maximal anteflexion to ensure good probe contact. This anteflexion should not be performed if resistance is encountered. From this position, rotation of

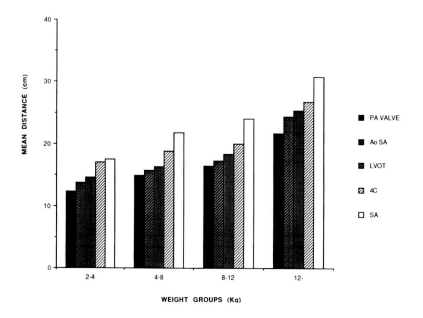

PA Valve - Pulmonary Artery, Ao SA - Aortic Short Axis, LVOT - Left Ventricular Outflow Tract, 4C - Four Chamber View, SA - Short Axis (Left Ventricle)

FIGURE 2–1. Distances that standard views are obtained from the central incisors or gums, according to weight. *PA valve,* pulmonic valve; *Ao sh,* aortic short axis view; *LVOT,* left ventricular outflow tract; *4C,* four-chamber view; *LV sh,* left ventricular short axis view. (*Reproduced with permission from Muhiudeen IA, et al. Echocardiography 10:599–608, 1993*)

the probe to the left with moderate flexion provides images of the anterior right ventricular outflow tract and the proximal pulmonary trunk as it courses anteriorly across the surface of the heart; rotation to the right and slight flexion from this position permit similar evaluation of the left ventricular outflow tract. Then the flexion of the probe is increased somewhat to define the inlet and outlet components of the ventricular septum as well as the atria and atrioventricular valves. The entrance of the pulmonary veins into the left atrium is demonstrated from this plane, and with rotation of the probe to the right the venoatrial connections of the right atrium can also be seen. Because the probe is some distance from the heart with a portion of the liver interposed, small movements of the transducer subtend large imaging arcs, permitting examination of the heart from the posterior atrial wall to near the anterior surface of the right ventricle. Following imaging of the outflow tracts, Doppler color flow mapping, pulsed and continuous-wave Doppler examinations, are performed from this transgastric location and from all other transducer locations as required by the suspected pathology.

Morphological Analysis

Assessment of the connections of the various cardiac segments, venoatrial, atrioventricular, and ventriculoatrial should be performed. Septal and valvar structures should then be evaluated, including as-

TABLE 2-1. COMPARATIVE DIAGNOSTIC UTILITY OF DEEP TRANSGASTRIC AND CONVENTIONAL TEE IMAGING

Atrial septal defects	Transverse TEE imaging provides better definition of ostium primum, ostium secundum compared to deep transgastric echocardiography. Deep transgastric echocardiography provides better definition of sinus venosus and anomalous pulmonary veins compared to transverse TEE.
Ventricular septal defects	Transverse TEE imaging displays perimembranous and muscular ventricular septal defects. TEE imaging and deep transgastric TEE define inlet ventricular septal defect well. TEE (longitudinal plane) provides better definition of outlet (doubly committed subaortic) ventricular septal defect.
Transposition	Deep transgastric echocardiography demonstrates the ventriculoarterial (simple and corrected) connections.
Truncus arteriosus	Deep transgastric echocardiography provides better definition of the ventriculoarterial connections compared to transverse TEE
Double inlet ventricles	Conventional and deep transgastric TEE displays atrioventricular connections well.
Double outlet ventricles	TEE and transgastric echocardiography define the ventriculoarterial connections well, but rotation of transesophageal echocardiography probe may visualize them as discordant.
Aortic stenosis (valvar and subvalvar)	Transgastric echocardiography provides good definition and continuous-wave Doppler estimates are easily obtained.
Atrioventricular septal defects	Transgastric echocardiography provides good definition of bridging leaflet and septal attachments.
Tetralogy of Fallot	Transgastric echocardiography provides better definition of aortic override and obstruction of the right ventricular outflow tract, the gradient for which is obtainable in 50% of patients.

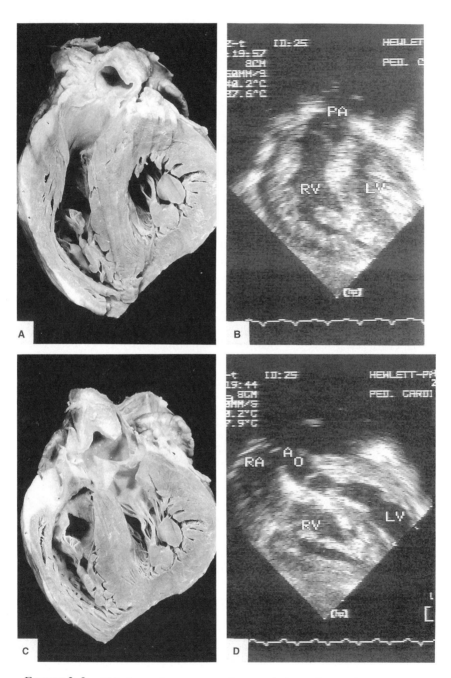

FIGURE 2–2. This figure demonstrates the morphology of the left and right ventricular outflow tracts from their respective ventricles with the corresponding cut specimens. (*A*) Anatomical specimen of the right ventricular outflow tract from the transgastric view, cut to display the morphology of an anteriorly di-

sessment of flow velocities with Doppler echocardiography. Both deep transgastric imaging and midesophageal longitudinal plane imaging accurately display the ventriculoarterial connections; our preference is the use of a deep transgastric approach because it has certain diagnostic advantages (Table 2–1).[16,17] This single-plane probe approach permits intraoperative imaging of the right and left ventricular outflow tracts from a vantage point similar to that achieved with the subcostal and subxyphoid precordial positions. To anatomically define deep transgastric imaging planes, slices were prepared from a normal heart (Figs. 2–2 and 2–3).[17] Representative deep transgastric images of individual lesions demonstrate the diagnostic value of this approach.

Recognition of Common Lesions

Tetralogy of Fallot

Aortic override is clearly demonstrated in the deep transgastric view (Figs. 2–4 and 2–5). A corresponding anatomical specimen cut in this plane reveals the ventricular septal defect, the aortic override, and the right ventricular hypertrophy (Fig. 2–4C), information also found with posteroanterior angiographic views. After surgical repair, the position of the patch and the increased size of the right ventricular outflow tract (Fig. 2–5) can be appreciated, as can relief of obstruction at the pulmonary infundibulum. Leaks around the patch (if present) can also be reliably detected.

Truncus Arteriosus Type 1

The common arterial trunk valve (TR), aorta (AO), and pulmonary arterial connections are clearly displayed from the deep transgastric

---

rected plane through the right ventricular outflow tract and the pulmonary artery. (*B*) Transgastric echocardiogram displaying a normal right ventricular outflow tract with the anterior papillary muscles and septomarginal trabeculation. The left ventricle is shown in its short axis. *PA*, pulmonary artery; *RV*, right ventricle; *LV*, left ventricle. (*C*) Anatomical specimen of the left ventricular outflow tract to simulate the transgastric view. This slice is posterior to the previous cut, showing the aorta arising from the left ventricle. The tricuspid valve is seen in the posterior inlet portion of the right ventricle. The mitral valve and its tendinous attachments are seen. (*D*) Transgastric echocardiogram of a left ventricular outflow tract showing the left ventricle and the ventriculoarterial connection to the aorta. The supravalvar aortic area is well displayed. *AO*, aorta; *RA*, right atrium. (*Reproduced with permission from Muhiudeen IA, et al. J Am Soc Echocardiogr 8:231–244, 1995*)

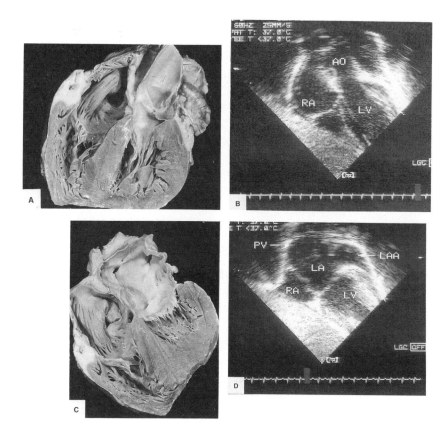

FIGURE 2–3. This figure demonstrates the morphology of the membranous and muscular components of the atrioventricular septum. (*A*) Anatomical specimen cut to display the atrioventricular component of the membranous septum (interposed between right atrium and subaortic outlet). (*B*) Corresponding transgastric echocardiogram displaying the membranous septum. *AO*, aorta; *RA*, right atrium; *LV*, left ventricle. (*C*) The most posterior cut in anatomical specimen revealing the musculoatrioventricular septum, inlet valves, and entrance of the pulmonary veins. (*D*) Transgastric echocardiogram demonstrating the inlet valves, left atrium, and a portion of the left atrial appendage. *LA*, left atrium; *LAA*, left atrial appendage; *PV*, pulmonary vein. (*Reproduced with permission from Muhiudeen IA, et al. J Am Soc Echocardiogr 8:231–244, 1995*)

plane in two patients with this lesion (Fig. 2–6A and B). Flexion and deflexion of the probe permit visualization of the truncal valve, its relation to the septum, the origins of the right and left pulmonary arteries (RPA, LPA), and the aorta from the common arterial trunk.

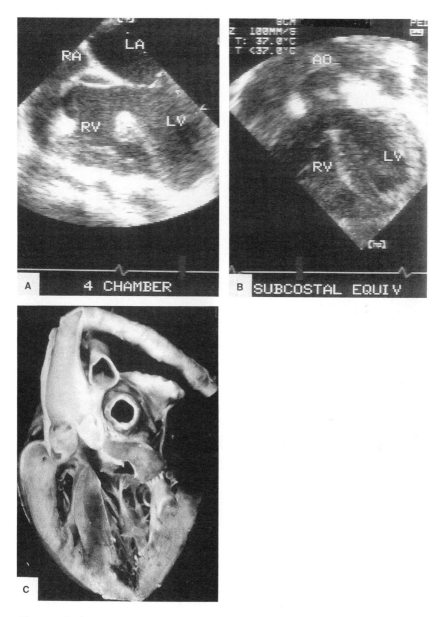

FIGURE 2-4. This figure demonstrates the morphology of a patient with tetralogy of Fallot and the corresponding transesophageal and transgastric echocardiograms. (*A*) Transesophageal four-chamber view in a patient with tetralogy of Fallot showing the override of the aorta. *LA*, left atrium; *LV*, left ventricle; *RA*, right atrium; *RV*, right ventricle. (*B*) Transgastric echocardiogram view showing the aortic override and ventricular septal defect in a case of tetralogy of Fallot (labeled subcostal view). *AO*, aorta. (*C*) Anatomical specimen of a patient with tetralogy of Fallot, displaying the right ventricular hypertrophy and the aorta overriding the ventricular septal defect. (*Reproduced with permission from Muhiudeen IA, et al. J Am Soc Echocardiogr 8:231–244, 1995*)

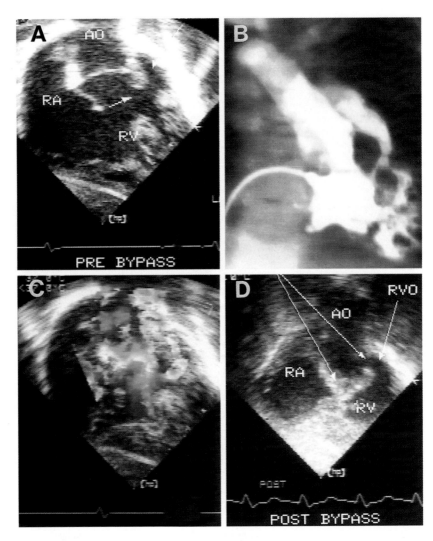

FIGURE 2–5. This figure demonstrates a patient with tetralogy of Fallot, comparing the transgastric echocardiogram to the corresponding angiogram, and flow through the ventricular septal defect out the right ventricular outflow tract. (A) Transgastric echocardiogram of the same patient with tetralogy of Fallot demonstrating the ventricular septal defect and aortic override. The right ventricular outflow tract is displayed anteriorly (*arrows*). AO, aorta; RA, right atrium; RV, right ventricle. (B) Corresponding angiogram in the same patient demonstrating the right ventricular outflow tract and the component of the subpulmonic stenosis. (C) Corresponding transgastric echocardiogram with color Doppler to show the flow through the ventricular septal defect, into the right ventricular outflow tract, and out through the pulmonary artery stenosis. (D) Transgastric echocardiogram after surgical repair showing placement of the patch (*arrows*) and right ventricular outflow tract. (*Reproduced with permission from Muhiudeen IA, et al. J Am Soc Echocardiogr 8:231–244, 1995*)

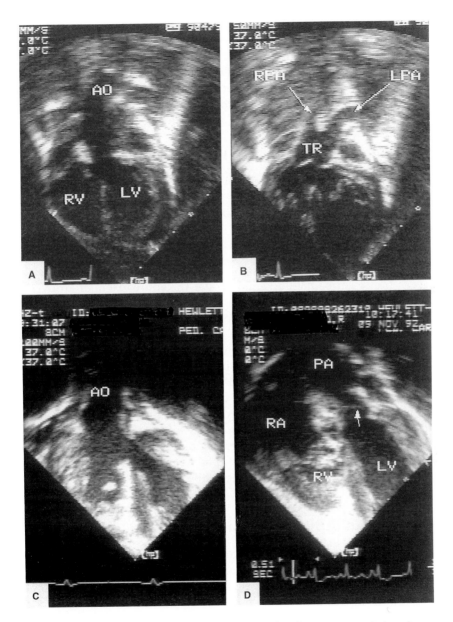

FIGURE 2–6. This figure demonstrates patients in whom transgastric imaging is necessary to demonstrate the ventriculoarterial connections, such as truncus arteriosus or transposition. (*A*) Transgastric echocardiogram of truncus arteriosus showing the ventriculoarterial connections with a large central vessel arising above the ventricular septal defect *AO*, aorta; *RV*, right ventricle; *LV*, left ventricle. (*B*) Transgastric echocardiogram of a second case of truncus arteriosus (type II) with origins of the right and left pulmonary artery (*RPA, LPA*) displayed clearly from a large common trunk *TR*, truncal vessel. (*C*) Transgastric

Legend continues on page 54.

Transposition of the Great Vessels

Deep transgastric imaging demonstrates the discordant ventriculoarterial connections (Fig. 2–6C and D) more clearly than the esophageal views, where the transposed great vessels can usually be visualized but the ventriculoarterial connections cannot.

Hypoplastic Left Heart Syndrome

The hypoplastic aortic root (AO) and the origins of the right and left coronary arteries (RCA, LCA) are well demonstrated relative to the normal sized pulmonary trunk (Fig. 2–7A and B).

Atrioventricular Septal Defect

Deep transgastric imaging demonstrates the entire extent of atrioventricular septal defects and the atrioventricular valve attachments. The interatrial communications (arrows) and entrance of the pulmonary veins into the left atrium (LA), and the morphology, type, and extension of the bridging leaflets can be imaged (Fig. 2–7C and D).

Representative echocardiograms of atrial and ventricular septal defects by transverse TEE are not presented in this chapter, because previous publications have amply documented that TEE imaging provides reliable images of these defects. The deep transgastric and other transverse planes provide complementary information for imaging the spectrum of ventricular septal defects, but lesions involving doubly committed subarterial ventricular septal defects are best imaged using the longitudinal plane of a biplane probe.[18–21]

Assessment of Pressure Gradients

The deep transgastric approach allows axial alignment for Doppler estimates of gradients across the outflow tracts and their quantitative assessment, thereby permitting intraoperative detection of residual ob-

---

echocardiogram in a case of simple transposition. The transposed aorta arises from the more anterior right-sided chamber with right ventricular morphology. There is a ventricular septal defect present. The *arrows* indicate origins of the coronary arteries. (*D*) Transgastric echocardiogram showing the pulmonary artery arising from the posterior left-sided chamber of left-sided morphology in a second case of transposition. *RA*, right atrium. (*Reproduced with permission from Muhiudeen IA, et al. J Am Soc Echocardiogr 8:231–244, 1995*)

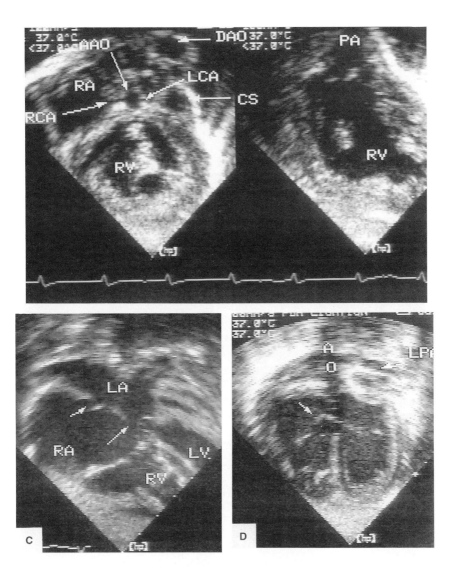

FIGURE 2–7. This figure demonstrates two congenital heart lesions displayed well by transgastric imaging, a hypoplastic left ventricle, and an atrioventricular septal defect. (*A*) Transgastric view of a case of hypoplastic left ventricle, with small aorta (*AO*) and coronary arteries (*RCA, LCA*) shown. The descending aorta (*DAo*) is also shown, along with the coronary sinus (*CS*). The pulmonary artery (*PA*) is of normal size. *RV*, right ventricle. (*B*) Transgastric imaging of the right ventricular outflow tract and normal sized pulmonary artery (*PA*) in the same patient. (*C*) Transgastric echocardiogram in a patient with atrioventricular septal defect, showing the interarterial septal defect (*arrow*) and the entrance of the pulmonary veins. *LA*, left atrium; *LV*, left ventricle; *RA*, right atrium. (*D*) Transgastric echocardiogram in a patient with atrioventricular septal defect, showing the muscular atrioventricular septum and free-floating (*LPA*, left pulmonary artery) bridging leaflets (*arrow*). (*Reproduced with permission from Muhiudeen IA, et al. J Am Soc Echocardiogr 8:231–244, 1995*)

structions.[17,22] This approach overcomes the limitations of transverse single-plane and biplane imaging of these structures. For example, biplane imaging with a longitudinal plane can visualize the right ventricular outflow tracts but provides only anatomical and color Doppler information; gradients cannot be assessed because of poor alignment of the Doppler beam with the direction of blood flow.

Doppler measurements of the right and left ventricular outflow gradients should be performed from the deep transgastric position (using the modified Bernoulli equation [peak pressure difference = 4 $(V)^2$]) (Figs. 2–8 and 2–9). In our series and others,[17,22] excellent agreement has been confirmed between Doppler estimates and direct pressure measurements. Thus, this technique can provide the operative team with an on-line assessment of pressure gradients before and after the surgical repair. Importantly the preoperative estimates of gradients

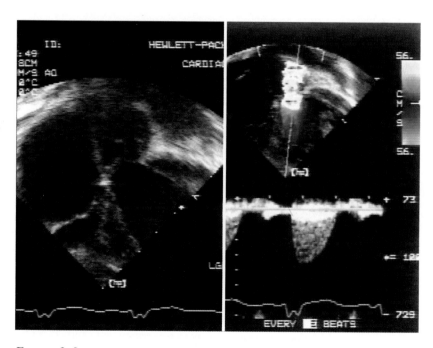

FIGURE 2–8. Transgastric echocardiogram of a patient with subaortic stenosis, demonstrating the fibrous ridge clearly from this plane (*left*). On the right, the flow disturbance caused by this condition is shown by Doppler flow imaging. Alignment of the continuous-wave cursor is demonstrated (*top right*). The *bottom right* continuous wave Doppler tracing shows an increase in velocity caused by this ridge. Scale markers are 0.2 seconds on the horizontal axis and 1-m/second intervals (vertical axis). (*Reproduced with permission from Muhiudeen IA, et al. J Am Soc Echocardiogr 8:231–244, 1995*)

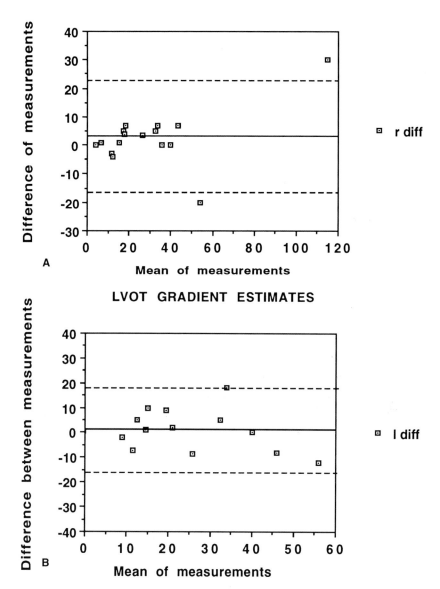

FIGURE 2–9. (*A and B*) Graphic display of the comparison of the difference in pressure gradients across the right and left ventricular outflow tracts derived by Doppler and cardiac catheterization or direct pressure gradient measurements. The vertical axis shows the difference between the measurements, and the horizontal axis presents the mean measurement obtained by each method. (*Reproduced with permission from Muhiudeen IA, et al. J Am Soc Echocardiogr 8:231–244, 1995*)

obtained when patients are lightly sedated may be different from those obtained by TEE at the time of operation.

COMPLICATIONS

Serious complications from TEE are very rare. However, hemodyamics and respiration must be closely monitored during TEE. Blood pressure generally remains stable but can drop precipitously if anteflexion or retroflexion compresses the aorta (Fig. 2–10). Therefore, we recommend placement of the TEE probe after arterial line placement.[11,23] Respiratory compromise can occur, peak inspiratory pressures can increase, and desaturation can take place. In addition, movement of the endotracheal tube during the TEE examination may occur, resulting in right mainstream intubation or extubation of the trachea. If desaturation suddenly occurs,[11,17,24,25] correct position must be confirmed, and sometimes the TEE probe must be immediately withdrawn. For all the above reasons, we recommend frequent nitoring of the peak inspiratory pressures throughout the TEE examinations.

CONTRAINDICATIONS

Recommendations have been made by the American Society of Echocardiography,[26] which were written for outpatient TEE. *Absolute contraindications* are unrepaired tracheoesophageal fistula, esophageal

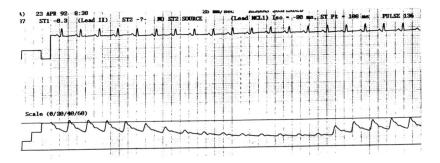

FIGURE 2–10. Graphic demonstration of hypotension during transesophageal echocardiographic examination. The electrocardiogram and arterial blood pressure tracing are displayed. (*Reproduced with permission from Roberson DA, et al. Echocardiogr 7:699–712, 1990*)

obstruction or stricture, perforated hollow viscus, active gastrointestinal bleeding, severe respiratory decompensation, or inadequate control of the airway. *Relative contraindications* include cervical spine injury or deformity, postesophageal surgery, esophageal varices or diverticulum, and oropharyngeal distortion or deformity.

ENDOCARDITIS PROPHYLAXIS

Endocarditis after TEE examinations has been reported, but usually when children are examined with TEE during surgery, antibiotics are routinely administered. In other situations antibiotic prophylaxis guidelines should follow those of the American Heart Association for endoscopy.[27]

CHANGES IN INTRAOPERATIVE SURGICAL MANAGEMENT

The overall incidence of change in surgical management due to intraoperative TEE is 7% in our series and others.[11,17,22] This incidence is not different from that reported with epicardial echocardiography.[1,7,10] Stevenson et al.[22] evaluated the surgical repair in 230 patients undergoing congenital heart surgery. After cardiopulmonary bypass, TEE prompted a return to bypass in 7.4% of their patients: 9 of 28 of these because of left ventricular outflow obstruction, 5 of 78 because of ventricular septal defects, and 3 of 51 because of other residual problems needing further surgery. All of their findings were confirmed by additional surgery. In conclusion, they stated that "TEE offers substantial utility in detection of residual problems requiring reoperation." Our results coincided with those of Stevenson et al.[22] and other centers.[7] In addition, our results suggested that with deep transgastric imaging of residual gradients, the need for return to bypass is discovered in an additional 2.2% of patients (Table 2–2). It is clear that TEE has significant perioperative impact in the care of infants and children undergoing surgical repair of congenital heart disease. The diagnoses are confirmed preoperatively, or if altered,[1,3,5,7] the surgical plan can be altered.[5,17,22] In order for the echocardiographer to perform a good complete postbypass echocardiographic examination, attention to specific detail with specific lesions should occur (Table 2–3). Reported residual lesions that can occur postcardiopulmonary bypass are shown in Figure 2–11.

TABLE 2–2. SURGICAL ALTERATIONS BASED ON TRANSESOPHAGEAL ECHOCARDIOGRAPHY

Preoperative Diagnosis	Intraoperative TEE Findings	Alteration
1. Double outlet right ventricle. Complete atrioventricular septal defect.	Turbulence noted in right ventricular outflow tract by transgastric imaging only. Obstruction of 40 mm Hg confirmed by intraoperative manometry.	Further augmentation of infundibulum with a pericardial patch.
2. Subaortic stenosis (discrete membrane) status post-ventricular septal defect closure.	Transgastric echocardiography demonstrated residual left ventricular outflow tract gradient of 30 mm Hg, confirmed by intraoperative manometry.	Reexploration showed that no further resection was possible.
3. Large ventricular septal defect, right ventricular outflow tract obstruction of the Tetralogy type.	Turbulence noted across right ventricular outflow tract by transgastric echocardiography with estimated gradient of 40 mm Hg. Prominent thrill over pulmonary artery.	Reexploration and subvalvar incision in right ventricular outflow tract. Resection of obstructing muscle bundle from trabecular marginal band. Final gradient less than 10 mm Hg.
4. Double inlet ventricle.	Transgastric echocardiography showed a 90-mm Hg gradient across the ventricular septal defect, confirmed by direct pullback.	Substantial resection of the septal muscle was performed. Final gradient less than 10 mm Hg.
5. Tetralogy of Fallot with pulmonary atresia, patent ductus-dependent pulmonary circulation, secundum atrial septal defect.	Initial weaning from bypass demonstrated normal hemodynamics but extremely low oxygen saturation. Transgastric echocardiography revealed right-to-left atrial shunt flow.	Bypass was reinstituted and atrial septal defect closed completely.

TABLE 2–3. ESSENTIAL POST-TEE CHECKLIST FOR VARIOUS DIAGNOSES[a]

Atrial septal defect	
Secundum	Intact patch, no residual leaks on color Doppler, no L → R or R → L shunting with contrast (transverse planes).
Primum	As above, some degree of mitral regurgitation (less than moderate) may be acceptable.
Sinus venosus	Intact patch, no residual leaks on color Doppler, no L → R or R → L shunting with contrast, no pulmonary venous inflow obstruction (transgastric and longitudinal plane).
Ventricular septal defect	
Perimembranous	No L → R shunting with contrast. No residual VSD (by color Doppler and pulsed-wave Doppler) (transverse plane).
Doubly committed subarterial (supracristal)	No residual VSD (longitudinal plane). No residual aortic insufficiency (transverse plane). No RVOT obstruction (deep transgastric plane).
Muscular, apical, inlet	No residual VSD as above (transverse and transgastric plane).
Atrioventricular septal defect	
Rastelli A, B, C (different levels of attachment of bridging leaflets)	No residual L or R atrioventricular valvar regurgitation (transverse and transgastric plane). Mild regurgitation may be acceptable. No residual ASD/VSD. No new VSDs (Fig. 2–11B).
Tetralogy of Fallot or pulmonic stenosis	No residual VSD (transverse plane). No residual RVOT obstruction or insufficiency (transgastric view).
Subaortic stenosis, aortic or supraaortic stenosis	No residual LVOT obstruction (transgastric view). No new VSD (Fig. 2–11A).
Arterial switch (Jatene procedure)	Evaluation of left ventricular function (transverse and longitudinal view). No significant segmental wall motion abnormalities. No significant AI or PI, no LVOT or RVOT obstruction (deep transgastric view).
Tricuspid atresia/Fontan procedure	Assessment of Fontan connection by pulsed wave Doppler[30]

Table 2-3 continues on page 62.

TABLE 2–3. ESSENTIAL POST-TEE CHECKLIST FOR VARIOUS DIAGNOSES[a] (Continued)

Double outlet right ventricle	Assessment of subaortic area and VSD patch (transgastric view).
Ross procedure	No residual (greater than mild) aortic or pulmonic stenosis or insufficiency (transgastric view). Evaluation of ventricular function (transverse view).

[a]ASD, atrial septal defect; VSD, ventricular septal defect; RVOT, right ventricular outflow tract; LVOT, left ventricular outflow tract; AI, aortic insufficiency; PI, pulmonic insufficiency.

INDICATIONS FOR INTRAOPERATIVE TEE

Documentation of Surgical Repair

TEE is indicated during repair of atrial and ventricular septal defects, atrioventricular septal defects, and tetralogy of Fallot. It is also indicated for valve repair and replacement and during surgery for obstructive lesions, such as subaortic and aortic stenosis and pulmonic stenosis. In other defects, such as patent ductus arteriosus and coarctation of the aorta, the potential risks (although small) may outweigh any potential benefit of TEE.

Assessment of Ventricular Function

TEE assesses global left ventricular function indirectly by measurement of cardiac output, stroke volume, or ejection fraction.[28] In addition, TEE can measure those factors that directly affect ventricular function: preload, contractility, and afterload. In particular, TEE has been shown to be a reliable monitor of cardiac filling changes in pediatric patients: in a recent study, in patients undergoing surgical repair of congenital heart lesions, blood was withdrawn until the systolic blood pressure decreased by 5 and 10 mm Hg.[29] Experienced anesthesiologist-echocardiographers blinded to study events were able to identify these mild reductions in blood volume by changes in left ventricular end diastolic afterload with high sensitivity (80 to 95%) and specificity (80%).

CONCLUSION

In many centers TEE is now the standard of care for intraoperative assessment of most congenital heart repairs prior to removal of bypass

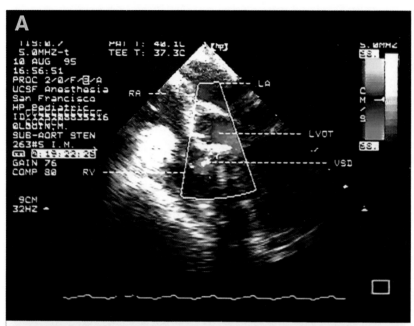

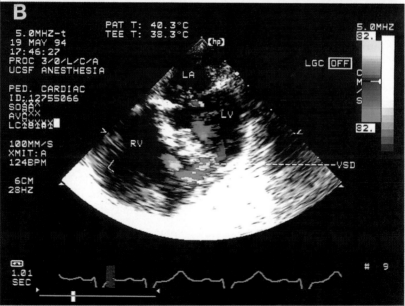

FIGURE 2-11. (*A*) Five-chamber view of a patient after resection of subaortic membrane showing newly created ventricular septal defect. *LA,* left atrium; *RA,* right atrium, *RV,* right ventricle; *LVOT,* left ventricular outflow tract; *VSD,* ventricular septal defect. (*B*) Four-chamber view of a patient after repair of atrioventricular septal defect showing apical muscular VSD not identified pre-operatively. *LV,* left ventricle.

cannulas and closure of the sternotomy. In addition, it provides a real-time method for assessment of ventricular function and volume status. It has become a valuable adjunct to the armamentarium of intraoperative anesthetic and surgical management.

References

1. Ungerleider RM, Kisslo JA, Greeley WJ: Intraoperative prebypass and postbypass epicardial color flow imaging in the repair of atrioventricular septal defects. J Thorac Cardiovasc Surg 98:90–100, 1989
2. Stumper O, Kaulitz R, Sreeram N, Fraser AG, Hess J, Roelandt JR, Sutherland GR: Intraoperative transesophageal versus epicardial ultrasound in surgery for congenital heart disease. J Am Soc Echocardiogr 3(5):392–401, 1990
3. Muhiudeen IA, Roberson DA, Silverman NH, Haas G, Turley K, Cahalan MK: Intraoperative echocardiography in infants and children with congenital cardiac shunt lesions: Transesophageal versus epicardial echocardiography. J Am Coll Cardiol 16(7):1687–1695, 1990
4. Ritter SB: Transesophageal echocardiography in children: New peephole to the heart. J Am Coll Cardiol 16(2):447–450, 1990
5. Muhiudeen IA, Roberson DA, Silverman NH, Haas GS, Turley K, Cahalan MK: Intraoperative echocardiography for evaluation of congenital heart defects in infants and children. Anesthesiology 76(2):165–172, 1992
6. Gussenhoven EJ, van HL, Roelandt J, Ligtvoet KM, Bos E, Witsenburg M: Intraoperative two-dimensional echocardiography in congenital heart disease. J Am Coll Cardiol 9(3):565–572, 1987
7. Ungerleider RM, Greeley WJ, Sheikh KH, Philips J, Pearce FB, Kern FH, Kisslo JA: Routine use of intraoperative epicardial echocardiography and Doppler color flow imaging to guide and evaluate repair of congenital heart lesions. A prospective study. J Thorac Cardiovasc Surg 100(2): 297–309, 1990
8. Roberson DA, Muhiudeen IA, Silverman NH, Turley K, Haas GS, Cahalan MK: Intraoperative transesophageal echocardiography of atrioventricular septal defect. J Am Coll Cardiol 18(2):537–545, 1991
9. Hsu YH, Santulli T Jr, Wong AL, Drinkwater D, Laks H, Williams RG: Impact of intraoperative echocardiography on surgical management of congenital heart disease. Am J Cardiol 67(15):1279–1283, 1991
10. Papagiannis J, Kanter RJ, Armstrong BE, Greeley WJ, Ungerleider RM: Intraoperative epicardial echocardiography during repair of tetralogy of fallot. J Am Soc Echocardiogr 6(4):366–373, 1993
11. Muhiudeen IA, Silverman NH: Transesophageal echocardiography using high resolution imaging in infants and children with congenital heart disease. Echocardiography 10:599–608, 1993
12. Greeley WJ, Ungerleider RM: Echocardiography during surgery for congenital heart disease. Intraoperative use of echocardiography: 129–155, 1991
13. Schiller NB, Maurer G, Ritter SB, Armstrong WF, Crawford M, Spotnitz H, Cahalan M, Quinones M, Meltzer R, Feinstein S: Transesophageal echocardiography. J Am Soc Echocardiogr 2(5):354–357, 1989
14. Seward JB, Khandheria BK, Oh JK, Abel MD, Hughes RJ, Edwards WD, Nichols BA, Freeman WK, Tajik AJ: Transesophageal echocardiography:

Technique, anatomic correlations, implementation, and clinical applications. Mayo Clin Proc 63(7):649–680, 1988

15. Bansal RC, Shah PM: Transesophageal echocardiography. Curr Probl Cardiol 15(11):641–720, 1990

16. Hoffman P, Stumper O, Rydelwska SW, Sutherland GR: Transgastric imaging: A valuable addition to the assessment of congenital heart disease by transverse plane transesophageal echocardiography. J Am Soc Echocardiogr 6(1):35–44, 1993

17. Muhiudeen IA, Silverman NH, Anderson RH: Transesophageal transgastric echocardiography in infants and children: The subcostal view equivalent. J Am Soc Echocardiogr 8:231–244, 1995

18. Ritter SB: Transesophageal real-time echocardiography in infants and children with congenital heart disease. J Am Coll Cardiol 18(2):569–580, 1991

19. Lam J, Neirotti RA, Lubbers WJ, Naeff MS, Blom-Muilwijk CM, Schuller JL, Macartney FJ, Visser CA: Usefulness of biplane transesophageal echocardiography in neonates, infants and children with congenital heart disease. Am J Cardiol 72(9):699–706, 1993

20. O'Leary PW, Hagler DJ, Seward JB, Tajik AJ, Schaff HV, Puga FJ, Danielson GK: Biplane intraoperative transesophageal echocardiography in congenital heart disease. Mayo Clin Proc 70(4):317–326, 1995

21. Seward JB: Biplane and multiplane transesophageal echocardiography: Evaluation of congenital heart disease. Am J Card Imaging 9(2):129–136, 1995

22. Stevenson JG, K. SG, M. GD, G. HD, A. RE: Left ventricular outflow tract obstruction: An indication for intraoperative transesophageal echocardiography. Am Soc Echocardiogr 6(5):525–535, 1993

23. Lunn RJ, Oliver WJ, Hagler DJ, Danielson GK: Aortic compression by transesophageal echocardiographic probe in infants and children undergoing cardiac surgery. Anesthesiology 77(3):587–590, 1992

24. Sorensen G, Stevenson G, Siebert J: The mechanism of airway obstruction during intraoperative transesophageal echo in infants. J Am Coll Cardiol 19(3):237A, 1992

25. Gilbert TB, Panico FG, McGill WA, Martin GR, Halley DG, Sell JE: Bronchial obstruction by transesophageal echocardiography probe in a pediatric cardiac patient. Anesth Analg 74(1):156–158, 1992

26. Fyfe DA, Ritter SB, Snider AR, Silverman NH, Stevenson JG, Sorensen G, Ensing G, Ludomirsky A, Sahn DJ, Murphy D, et al: Guidelines for transesophageal echocardiography in children [see comments]. J Am Soc Echocardiogr 5(6):640–644, 1992

27. Dajani AS, Bisno AL, Chung KJ, Durack DT, Freed M, Gerber MA, Karchmer AW, Millard HD, Rahimtoola S, Shulman ST, et al: Prevention of bacterial endocarditis. Recommendations by the American Medical Association. JAMA 264(22):2919–2922, 1990

28. Matsumoto M, Oka Y, Lin YT, Strom J, Sonnenblick EH, Frater RW: Transesophageal echocardiography; for assessing ventricular performance. N Y State J Med 79(1):19–21, 1979

29. Reich DL, Konstadt SN, Nejat M, Abrams HP, Bucek J: Intraoperative transesophageal echocardiography for the detection of cardiac preload changes induced by transfusion and phlebotomy in pediatric patients. Anesthesiology 79(1):10–15, 1993

30. Stumper O, Sutherland GR, Geuskens R, Roelandt JR, Bos E, Hess J: Transesophageal echocardiography in evaluation and management after a Fontan procedure. J Am Coll Cardiol 17(5):1152–1160, 1991

Frank H. Kern
Scott Schulman
William J. Greeley

Cardiopulmonary Bypass: Techniques and Effects

3

The development of a pump oxygenator for cardiac surgery was first pioneered by John Gibbon in the late 1930s, but a clinically useful device was not achieved for nearly 20 years. In the interim period, surgery on the human heart was severely limited. The length and quality of life for children with simple and complex congenital cardiac defects were dictated by the natural history of the disease process throughout the 1930s and mid-1940s. The introduction of palliative extracardiac shunting procedures (Blalock-Taussig, Potts' shunts) were introduced in the mid-1940s to extend life expectancy.[1,2] Yet despite palliation, life expectancy for these more complex cardiac defects remained poor. It was not until the genesis of circulatory support devices, i.e., cross-circulation techniques and true heart–lung machines, and the development of more modern operative and anesthetic techniques did the repair of complex cardiac defects become feasible. Demonstrable improvements in life expectancy and quality followed the introduction of these important developments of the 1950s and 1960s.

In the 1950s, techniques to preserve organ function and allow operative procedures to be performed on the heart without cardiopulmonary bypass (CPB) were pioneered by Bigelow.[3,4] Bigelow described the experimental use of deep hypothermia using a topical ice bath as a method for preserving organ function in a canine model. Circulatory arrest for periods of up to 15 minutes were well tolerated.

Perioperative Management of the Patient with Congenital Heart Disease, edited by William J. Greeley. Williams & Wilkins, Baltimore © 1996.

After experimental success in the dog, several investigators used similar surface cooling techniques to repair atrial septal defects (ASDs) in children.[4,5] Although this technique provided brief periods for surgical correction, surface cooling techniques were problematic. Systemic hypotension, brady- and tachydysrhythmias, coagulopathies, acid–base imbalance, and limited operative periods of 15 minutes made the technique less than satisfactory. Only simple intracardiac defects, such as ASDs were successfully repaired using this approach.

In 1953, John Gibbon performed the first successful open-heart operation, a closure of an ASD in a young woman using a heart–lung machine.[6] The machine was large, cumbersome, and quite crude. It required 14 units of blood to prime and was fraught with a vast array of technical problems, including frequent and difficult to repair circuit disruptions, poor control of the patient's circulating blood volume, wide variation in perfusion flow rates, and an inability to monitor or maintain blood gases in a physiological range. Although the initial patient survived, subsequent patients did not, diminishing interest in this early device.

At the University of Minnesota, C. Walton Lillehei performed the first closure of a ventricular septal defect (VSD) using the technique of cross-circulation.[7] Cross-circulation was a novel technique requiring a human volunteer (usually a parent) to function as the circulatory support device for the surgical patient. A venous cannula was placed into the heart patient's superior vena cava and blood coursed through a pump head and into the femoral vein of the donor. A second cannula was placed into the donor's femoral artery, and flow from the femoral artery was returned to the heart patient's carotid artery. Forty-five patients, mostly children, were operated on using this technique beginning in 1954, and 63% of the patients survived, which was remarkable for the mid-1950s.[7,8] Cross-circulation, although an extremely novel and successful approach, was not a long-term solution for open cardiac procedures, because the human volunteer and the heart patient were placed at high risk of injury and/or death. It did prove, however, that open cardiac procedures could be performed successfully with cardiorespiratory support systems and fostered the continued development of pump oxygenator technology.

In the early 1950s, John Kirklin, then at the Mayo Clinic, began an intensive research effort to develop a clinically functional pump oxygenator based on the original work of Gibbon. After 2 years of successful laboratory work, eight children were selected for open-heart surgery using the Gibbon-Mayo pump oxygenator; four patients survived. The Gibbon-Mayo pump oxygenator required 5 to 11 units of freshly drawn blood to prime and required a slow controlled flow of blood through the oxygenator. This technique was necessary because blood foaming resulted in lethal emboli, and defoaming agents were unknown at this time.[9] Although crude, this device allowed total cardiorespiratory support for patients requiring operative procedures on the heart and ushered in a new era in pediatric cardiac surgery.

Since the 1950s, pediatric CPB has evolved from this high-risk technology with a 50% mortality into a safe and effective procedure performed at many hospitals throughout the world. Yet despite the success and nearly 40 years of investigation, the effect of CPB on the patient remains poorly understood. This is particularly true in children, were CPB technology remains an extreme departure from normal physiology.

DIFFERENCES OF PEDIATRIC VS ADULT BYPASS

The management of CPB in neonates, infants, and children differs substantially from the adult. Pediatric patients are exposed to biological extremes, including deep hypothermia (15 to 20°C), hemodilution (3 to 4-fold dilution of circulating blood volume), low perfusion pressures (20 to 30 mm Hg), wide variation in pump flow rates (ranging from highs of 200 ml/kg/minute to deep hypothermic circulatory arrest [DHCA]) and wide ranging blood pH management, e.g., controlled (alpha stat, pH stat) and uncontrolled (post-DHCA or post-low flow CPB, when pH can be extremely and unpredictably low). These CPB management parameters alter autoregulatory function. In addition to these prominent changes, subtle variations in glucose supplementation, cannula placement, presence of aortopulmonary collaterals, patient age, and size may also impair effective perfusion during CPB.

Adult patients are rarely, if ever, exposed to these biological extremes. Temperature is rarely lowered below 25°C, hemodilution is more moderate, perfusion pressure is generally maintained at 30 to 80 mm Hg, flow rates are maintained at 50 to 65 ml/kg/minute, and pH management strategy is less influential because moderate hypothermic temperatures are commonly used, whereas deep hypothermia and circulatory arrest are rarely used (Table 3–1). Variables such as glucose requirements and patient size are more consistent in adults. Venous and arterial cannulas are larger and less deforming of the atria and aorta, and their placement is more predictable. Although superficially similar, the conduct of CPB in children is considerably different from adults. Therefore, one would expect marked physiological differences in the response to CPB of the child in general and in particular of neonates and young infants.

TABLE 3–1. DIFFERENCES BETWEEN ADULT AND PEDIATRIC CPB

Parameter	Adult	Pediatric
Hypothermic temperature	Rarely below 25–32°C	Commonly 15–20°C
Use of total circulatory arrest	Rare	Common
Pump prime		
Effects of dilution on blood volume	25–33%	200–300%
Additional additives in pediatric primes		Blood, albumin
Perfusion pressures	50–80 mm Hg (some centers accept 30 mm Hg)	20–50 mm Hg
Influence of blood gas management strategy on measured PaCO$_2$	Minimal at moderate hypothermia	Marked at deep hypothermia
Alpha stat/pH stat	30 mm Hg/45 mm Hg	20 mm Hg/80 mm Hg
Glucose regulation		
Hypoglycemia	Rare—requires significant hepatic injury	Common—reduced hepatic glycogen stores
Hyperglycemia	Frequent—generally easily controlled with insulin	Less common—rebound hypoglycemia may occur

HYPOTHERMIC CPB: APPLICATION AND FUNCTION

The CPB circuit must replace the function of both the heart and lungs during cardiac surgery. Because of the use of nonpulsatile flow and the need for reduced perfusion flow rates to minimize blood return to the heart, hypothermia is required. Specifically, hypothermic CPB is used to preserve organ function during cardiac surgery and prevent end organ ischemia through a reduction in cellular metabolism and preservation of high-energy phosphate "stores." As temperature is lowered, both basal and functional cellular metabolism is reduced, and the rate of ATP and phosphocreatine consumption is substantially reduced.[10,11] At deep hypothermia, cellular metabolism is so low and membrane fluidity reduced to such a large extent that cellular basal metabolic needs and cellular membrane integrity can be maintained for a relatively prolonged period of time. This is the basis of the protective effects of deep hypothermia and allows for the implementation of low-flow deep hypothermic CPB and DHCA.

The degree of hypothermia selected is dependent on the need for reduced flow to enhance surgical repair. Three distinct methods of CPB are used: moderate hypothermia (25 to 32°C), deep hypothermia (15 to 20°C), or deep hypothermia with an interposed period of circulatory arrest (DHCA). The technique selected is based on the required surgical conditions, patient size, the type of operation, and the potential physiological impact on the patient.

Moderate hypothermic CPB is the principal method of bypass employed for older children and adolescents. In these patients, venous cannulas are less obtrusive and the heart can easily accommodate superior and inferior vena cava cannulation. Bicaval cannulation reduces right atrial blood return and improves the surgeon's ability to visualize intracardiac anatomy. The large cannulas used in older children are rigid and less likely to kink. Moderate hypothermia may also be chosen for less demanding cardiac repairs in infants, such as an ASD or uncomplicated VSD. Most surgeons are willing to cannulate the inferior vena cava (IVC) and superior vena cava (SVC) in neonates and infants. However, in neonates and infants this is technically more difficult and likely to induce brief periods of hemodynamic instability. Additionally, the pliability of the cava and the rigidity of the cannulas may result in caval obstruction, reduced venous drainage, and elevated venous pressure in the mesenteric and cerebral circulation. When moderate hypothermia is used, perfusion flow rates must be high to meet metabolic demands of the patient. Recommendations for optimal pump flow rates for children are based on the patients' body mass and maintaining efficient organ perfusion as determined by arterial blood gases, acid–base balance, and whole body oxygen consumption during CPB.[12,13] Table 3–2 lists recommended, albeit arbitrary, normothermic flow rates for children based on body weight. At hypothermic temperatures metabolism is reduced, and therefore pump flow rates may be further reduced. A discussion of low-flow CPB is presented later in this chapter.

Deep hypothermic CPB is generally reserved for neonates and infants requiring complex cardiac repairs. However, certain older children with complex cardiac disease or severe aortic valve regurgitation may benefit from deep hypothermic temperatures. For the most part, deep hypothermia is selected to allow the surgeon to operate under conditions of low-flow CPB or deep hypothermic circulatory arrest. Low pump flows improve the operating conditions for the surgeon by providing a near bloodless field and generally allow the use of a single atrial cannula resulting in better visualization of atrial anatomy and operative repairs performed through a right atriotomy.

Deep hypothermic CPB with deep hypothermic circulatory arrest allows the surgeon to remove the atrial and if necessary the aortic cannulas. Utilizing this technique, surgical repair is more precise because of the bloodless and cannula-free operative field. Arresting the circulation even at deep hypothermic temperatures introduces the question of how well deep hypothermia preserves organ function, with the brain being of greatest concern. Extensive clinical experience using DHCA has suggested the duration of a safe circulatory arrest period to be approximately 45 to 60 minutes. More formalized neurological investigation in neonates undergoing circulatory arrest suggests that arrest times of greater than 30 minutes may predispose patients to mild neurological deficits. Neurological impairment is more likely if a VSD is present and the patient is exposed to a period of DHCA. This suggests that systemic air embolism in conjunction with DHCA has a more than additive effect on neurological outcome.

TABLE 3–2. RECOMMENDED PUMP
FLOW RATES FOR CPB
IN CHILDREN

Patient Weight (kg) (ml/kg/min)	Pump Flow Rate
<3	150–200
3–10	125–175
10–15	120–150
15–30	100–120
30–50	75–100
>50	50–75

Although circulatory arrest may be harmful to the brain, it is well tolerated by other organs. Organ protection during the arrest period is a function of hypothermia and reduced exposure to the inflammatory response associated with exposure to the extracorporeal circuit. Hypothermia preserves organ function by maintaining cellular adenosine triphosphate (ATP) stores despite reduced delivery, by reducing glutamate release, and by preventing calcium entry into the cell even though energy-dependent calcium pumps are depleted of ATP stores. In addition, the myocardium, the lungs, and the body as a whole are protected from the inflammatory response associated with exposure to the extracorporeal circuit. The reduced exposure to cytokine release, complement activation, and total body water accumulation may preserve organ function.

PATHOPHYSIOLOGICAL CONSIDERATIONS OF CPB IN CHILDREN

Pathophysiological changes that occur during and after pediatric CPB relate to the nonendothelialized bypass circuit and oxygenator, hypothermia, the degree of hemodilution, nonpulsatile perfusion, the age of the patient, the preoperative myocardial substrate, the length of the ischemic period on the myocardium (cross-clamp time) or the entire body (deep hypothermic circulatory arrest time), the type of anesthesia used, and the exaggerated inflammatory response present in the young child. The effects on the patient are both global and organ specific. Global hormonal and metabolical responses have been characterized as the "stress response" to hypothermic CPB.

Global Effects of CPB

Stress Response and CPB

The release of a large number of metabolical and hormonal substances, including catecholamines, cortisol, growth hormone, prostaglandins, complement, interleukins and cytokines, glucose, insulin, β-endorphins, and other substances characterize the stress response during hypothermic CPB.[14–16] The likely causes for the elaboration of these substances include: contact of blood with the nonendothelialized surface of the pump tubing and oxygenator[17] nonpulsatile flow, low perfusion pressure, hemodilution, hypothermia, and reduced anesthetic depth. Other factors that may contribute to elevations of stress hormones include delayed renal and hepatic clearance during hypothermic CPB, myocardial injury, and exclusion of the pulmonary circulation from bypass. The lung is responsible for metabolizing and clearing many of these stress hormones. The stress response generally peaks during rewarming from CPB. There is evidence that the hormonal component of the stress response can be blunted but not eliminated by increasing the depth of anesthesia, especially using high-dose narcotics.[16,18]

It is unclear at what level elevated circulating stress hormones, normally an adaptive response, become detrimental. There is little question that these substances do mediate undesirable effects, such as myocardial damage (catecholamines), systemic and pulmonary hypertension (catecholamines), pulmonary endothelial damage (complement, interleukins, prostaglandins), and pulmonary vascular reactivity (thromboxane, interleukins). Recently, the benefits of ablation of the release of stress hormones and catecholamines with fentanyl in premature infants undergoing PDA ligation have been demonstrated. Additionally, neonates with complex congenital heart disease (CHD) who die in the postoperative period demonstrate much higher hormonal and metabolical responses during the intra- and postoperative periods compared to survivors with similar cardiac defects.[16,18] Although blunting the extremes of the stress hormone response seems warranted, there is additional evidence suggesting that the newborn stress response, especially the endogenous release of catecholamines, may be an adaptive metabolical response necessary for survival at birth.[19] This suggests that complete elimination of an adaptive stress response may not be desirable; however, modification of its extremes probably is. To what extent acutely ill neonates with CHD are dependent on their stress response for maintaining hemodynamic stability during and after CPB is currently unknown. Perhaps distinguishing maladaptive stress hormone release from adaptive release is the presence of mediators of systemic inflammation and endothelial injury.

Systemic Inflammation and Endothelial Injury

Complement activation, neutrophil activation, release and activation of tumor necrosis factor, and interleukins 1, 6, and 8 have been described during hypothermic CPB.[20-23] These mediators of systemic inflammation in conjunction with ischemia/reperfusion injury, hemodilution, and the direct effects of hypothermia account for widespread organ injury during and after CPB. The main target of many of these mediators is the vascular endothelium. Endothelial injury results in altered microcirculatory function which is responsible for elevations in pulmonary, cerebral, and systemic vascular resistance, a common finding after hypothermic CPB. Endothelial injury impairs release of important vasodilators, such as nitric oxide and prostacy-clin, and promotes release of vasoconstrictors such as thromboxane A_2 and endothelin (also known to have inotropic effects in the myocardium).[17,24–32] In addition to these properties, the endothelial surface (pulmonary endothelium in particular) is responsible for metabolizing vasoconstrictors such as angiotensin, catecholamines, and eicosanoids. Injured endothelium by virtue of reduced production of nitric oxide and impaired metabolism of mediators of vasodilators promotes vasoconstriction.[33] Endothelial cells also play an important regulatory role in water and solute transport. Abnormalities in endothelial function promote increased capillary permeability and increases in interstitial edema.

Nonpulsatile Perfusion

Evidence for microcirculatory dysfunction with nonpulsatile perfusion can be found in a large number of studies. Ogata and associates in 1960 directly observed that capillary flow in the momentum slowed and virtually ceased during nonpulsatile CPB at normothermia.[34] At flow rates of 60 and 75 ml/kg/minute, nonpulsatile flow resulted in lower total body oxygen consumption and lower pH and base deficits than with pulsatile perfusion. Matsumato et al. showed that at 37°C, nonpulsatile perfusion produced capillary sludging, dilation of the postcapillary venules, and increased edema formation in the conjunctival and cerebral microcirculation.[35]

In contrast, pulsatile CPB maintained capillary blood flow in the omentum, eliminated sludging in the conjunctival and cerebral microcirculation, and reduced jugular venous lactate levels.[34–36] Evidence also suggests that pulsatile perfusion may provide better cerebral perfusion. Studies of hypothermic low-flow CPB in a dog model demonstrate that converting low-flow nonpulsatile CPB at 25 ml/kg/minute to pulsatile perfusion improves brain pH, PCO_2, and PO_2.[37] Measurements of brain metabolism ($CMRO_2$) in neonates, infants, and children demonstrate that nonpulsatile perfusion accounts for a 9% reduction in brain metabolism.[38] Pulsatile perfusion may, therefore, improve cerebral perfusion at both normothermic and hypothermic temperatures. When low-flow CPB is used, the addition of pulsatile flow may provide improved microcirculatory perfusion and allow for better oxygen delivery to tissue at lower flow rates.

Mechanistically a lack of pulsatility alters the biomechanical forces exerted on the endothelium.[39,40] This results in rather rapid changes in ionic conductance, adenylate cyclase activity, and intracellular free calcium levels, similar to receptor-mediated changes in vascular tone seen with α- and β-receptors. If more prolonged exposure to nonpulsatile flow exists, changes in vascular tone may be augmented by release of local regulatory hormones, such as endothelin. These changes require alterations in gene expression.

Although improvements in microvascular flow and organ metabolism have been suggested with the addition of pulsatile flow, clinical studies have been inconclusive. Murkin and Farrar observed a 13% improvement in cerebral blood flow and cerebral oxygen consumption with pulstile CPB in adults.[41] Louagie and colleagues found no demonstrable improvement in physiological data, fluid balance, or clinical outcome variables in 100 adult coronary artery patients undergoing pulatile vs nonpusatile CPB.[42] In children, a small clinical trial of pulsatile CPB demonstrated no improvement in glucose, insulin, and cortisol responses during CPB.[43] Although trials have been limited, it appears that the benefits of pulsatile perfusion would be in patients with limited organ reserve or those exposed to more extreme perfusion variables such as low-flow CPB or DHCA. Clinical assessment of pulsatile perfusion during low-flow CPB or DHCA in the pediatric patient has as yet not been adequately evaluated.

Systemic Blood Flow and Metabolism during Hypothermic CPB

During high-flow hypothermic CPB, peripheral vascular resistance increases in all vascular beds throughout the body. Flow to the kidneys, gastrointestinal tract, and brain are decreased, and flow is preferentially shunted toward skeletal muscle.[44] This is quite different from the intact subject not exposed to CPB, who demonstrates an increase in peripheral vascular resistance and preferential flow to the brain, heart, and kidneys in response to a decrease in cardiac output. This difference between the hypothermic patient on and off CPB is dependent on the effects of hypothermia on cardiac output. In the canine surface cooled (without CPB) from 37° to 25°C, a 75% reduction in cardiac output (2.3 liters/min to 0.575 liter/min) was observed.[45] This marked reduction in cardiac output must be compensated by an increase in systemic vascular resistance. During hypothermic CPB when flow rates are maintained by the pump at high perfusion rates (flow rates of 3.01 liters/min), blood is shunted away from the vital organs to the skeletal muscle. The vasculature of skeletal muscle serves as a large capacitance bed for excessive flow during high-flow hypothermic CPB. During low-flow hypothermic CPB, skeletal muscle vasculature constricts and total body blood flow is redistributed toward vital organs. Vital organ blood flow is maintained and provides effective oxygen delivery to maintain identical oxygen consumption at both full flow and after a 50% reduction in perfusion flow rates.[44] In patients with aortopulmonary shunts, a common finding in cyanotic patients undergoing CPB, there is a greater redistribution of blood flow away from the gastrointestinal tract and kidneys.[46] This excessive shunting may contribute to the higher incidence of end-organ injury observed in infants with large aortopulmonary shunts or aortopulmonary collaterals when exposed to prolonged periods of CPB. Many centers attempt to coil large collateral vessels in the cardiac catheterization laboratory prior to surgery in an attempt to reduce shunt flow during CPB.

CO_2 Management: Alpha Stat and pH Stat

The role of CO_2 management in CPB has been studied extensively in animals and adult patients. Based on the effect of CO_2 on arterial and intracellular pH at hypothermic temperatures, two divergent blood gas management strategies have been championed: alpha stat (temperature uncorrected) and pH stat (temperature corrected).[11,12,47-50] Alpha-stat strategy maintains a pH of 7.40 measured without mathematical correction for the effects of temperature, whereas pH stat uses a mathematical correction for the effects of temperature on pH. With temperature-corrected measurements, blood pH becomes increasingly alkalotic as the blood cools. To correct for this alkalotic "pH," CO_2 is added to maintain a temperature-corrected pH of 7.40 (pH stat). The addition of CO_2, however, lowers *intracellular* pH (pHi) resulting in an imbalance between H^+ and OH^- ions, i.e., the loss of electrochemical neutrality. Intracellular enzymatic function depends on maintaining a normal pHi, and therefore cellular enzyme function may be impaired using pH stat. An acidotic pHi is increasingly problematic because at hypothermic temperatures the normal buffering systems (NH_3^-, HCO_3^-) become ineffective. At hypothermia, buffering capacity is limited to negative charges of the amino acids composing intracellular proteins. The amino acid histidine is the most important buffer at hypothermia because it contains an α-imidazole ring with many negatively charged moieties that can buffer H^+ ions. The reason uncorrected blood gas measurement is called "alpha" stat is in reference to the imadizole ring of histidine. The principal advantage of alpha-stat strategy, therefore, is preserving intracellular electrochemical neutrality, maintaining appropriate intracellular pH (pHi), and improving the efficiency of intracellular enzymatic function.[51] More recently the alterations in intracellular pH associated with pH stat management has been questioned. Work by Aoki et al. and Swain et al. using (NMR) techniques suggests minimal change in intracellular pH during pH stat. These data suggest that pH stat may not have a deleterious effect on intracellular pH as previously thought. However, the effect of tissue pH or more precisely the pH of the microcirculation is acidotic. This may have a deleterious effect on microcirculatory function and the ability of the microcirculation to effectively deliver oxygen to tissue.[52,53]

Systemic Air Embolism during Hypothermic CPB

During CPB, microembolic events commonly occur and can contribute to end-organ injury.[54,55] Air and particulate emboli have been demonstrated by middle cerebral artery transcranial Doppler, retinal angiography, echocardiography, direct visualization of coronary vessels, and by electrocardiographic analysis.[56–60] Neurological events have been correlated with the presence of focal dilatations of the microvasculature or very small aneurysms in terminal arterioles and capillaries within the cerebral circulation.[57] The use of membrane oxygenators, arterial filters, and adequate heparinization (ACT >400 sec) during CPB decreases the number of microemboli and may reduce the incidence of embolic events during CPB.[60–62] Yet, despite these methods, air embolism remains an important factor in postoperative neurological dysfunction. During pediatric CPB, the frequency in which the left side of the circulation is exposed to air increases the likelihood of systemic air embolization. In a recent report of perioperative neurological effects in neonates undergoing the arterial switch operation for transposition of the great arteries, the presence of a VSD was associated with an increased incidence of postoperative seizure activity and psychomotor dysfunction.[63] This strongly suggests air embolism as an etiology for neurological dysfunction.

Intramyocardial air has also been suggested as a contributing factor for right ventricular dysfunction after pediatric cardiac surgery.[58,64] In 4% of 350 consecutive pediatric patients undergoing repair of congenital cardiac defects, intramyocardial air was detected in the immediate postbypass period using echocardiography with Doppler imaging.[58] Echo-Doppler demonstrated increased echogenic areas localized to the right ventricular free wall and along the inferior portion of the intraventricular septum. Hemodynamic instability was a significant finding in many of these patients. The distribution of air was localized to the area supplied by the right coronary artery. The right coronary artery is a likely source for embolization of retained left ventricular air because of the location of the ostium of the right coronary artery on the anterior aspect of the aorta. Therefore, residual left ventricular air is more likely to enter the right coronary artery and result in right ventricular ischemia and dysfunction.

Therapy for air embolism is directed at increasing perfusion pressure to propel air through the arterioles and capillary bed. Dramatic hemodynamic and echocardiographic improvements have been demonstrated in patients with intramyocardial air after the administration of phenylephrine or reperfusing the heart with high pump flow rates and perfusion pressures on CPB[58] (Fig. 3–1). This approach can also be utilized in patients with cerebral air emboli. Alternatively, cerebral air embolism can be approached by reducing gas bubble size either by reestablishing hypothermic CPB or through the use of hyperbaric oxygen therapy in the early postoperative period.[65,66] Both hypothermia and hyperbaric therapy reduce the size of gaseous microbubbles and allow them to pass through the arterial and capillary beds resulting in reduced tissue damage.

Organ-Specific Effects of Hypothermic CPB

Myocardial Effects

General Considerations of the Neonatal Heart

The neonatal heart appears to be more resistant to ischemic and reperfusion injury than the normal adult heart. Much of this protection is due to a resistance to calcium influx during and after an ischemic event and larger energy stores in immature myocytes. Calcium influx is reduced by the sarcolemma of the immature heart which binds calcium more avidly then mature myocardium, thereby reducing calcium entry and calcium-induced cellular injury.[67] In addition, the immature myocardium, by virtue of its growth requirements, has increased glycogen and amino acid stores which increases cellular anaerobic and aerobic capacity when nutrient delivery is reduced by ischemia.[68,69,70] These factors appear to protect the normal immature myocardium from ischemic injury.

Exposure to hemodiluted perfusion, however, is poorly tolerated by the neonatal myocardium.[71] Mavroudis and Ebert demonstrated a significant worsening in myocardial compliance in neonatal hearts exposed to hemodiluted perfusate. Nonhemodiluted perfusate did not alter left ventricular compliance in the neonate, and hemodilution had minimal effect on left ventricular compliance in adult hearts.

The cyanotic neonate or the neonate who presents in congestive failure appears to have a myocardial substrate which is less tolerant of ischemia than the normal neonatal heart.[72] Experimental evidence suggests that this is most likely due to impaired substrate delivery

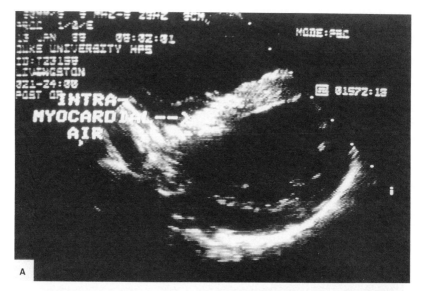

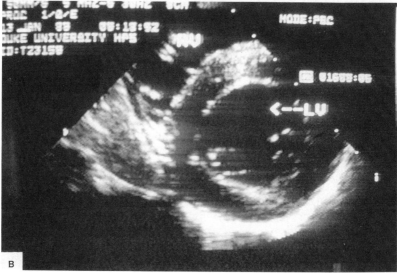

FIGURE 3-1. (A) Two-dimensional echocardiogram recorded in the short-axis view using an epicardial approach demonstrates intramyocardial air localized to the ventricular septum and the right ventricular free wall. The ventricular septum is flattened, depicting abnormal septal motion. (B) Phenylephrine was administered to increase coronary artery perfusion pressure. A repeat two-dimensional echocardiogram shows resolution of the echogenic region in the septum and right ventricular free wall and a normal left ventricular dimension.

and marginal myocardial energy reserves.[72,73] Neonatal hearts also have a reduced response to exogenous administration of β-agonists. Dobutamine in doses of 6 to 20 μg/kg/minute results in only a modest increase in load-independent measures of contractility. In contrast, propranolol results in a severe reduction in load-independent measures of contractility. This suggests that reduced β-receptor number and high-circulation catecholamines result in a maximal β-adrenoceptor binding in neonatal animals at rest.

Effects of CPB on Myocardial Receptor Function

CPB also desensitizes cardiac β-receptors. Schwinn and colleagues examined the effects of β-agonists on adenyl cyclase activity in canine left ventricular tissue.[74] Maximal isoproterenol stimulation resulted in a marked increase in β-receptor-mediated adenyl cyclase activity in the pre-CPB period. After 155 minutes of CPB, reexposure to the same isoproterenol dose resulted in a significant decrease in β-receptor-stimulated adenyl cyclase activity. Thirty minutes after bypass adenyl cyclase activity was equal to or greater than prebypass measurements (Fig. 3–2). Similar responses where obtained when submaximal infu-

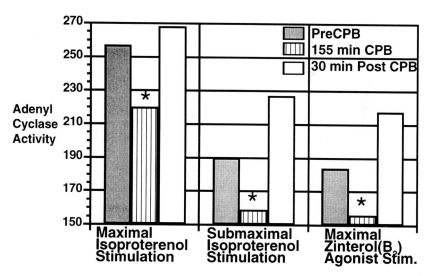

FIGURE 3–2. A bar graph depicting the effects of CPB on cardiac β-adrenergic receptors during CPB in the dog. Adenyl cyclase activity is measured from left ventricular transmyocardial biopsy specimens taken pre-CPB, during CPB, and 30 minutes post-CPB. Significant decreases in beta-stimulated adenyl cyclase activity were documented after CPB when compared with pre- and post-CPB values. The beta-specific drugs used were isoproterenol (100-μM and 500-nM concentrations) and zinterol (100-μM), a β_2-specific drug. *, $P < .05$.

sions of isoproterenol and the β_2-selective drug, zinterol, were used. When β-receptor density was examined, it was found to be unchanged during CPB, suggesting that the reduction in function related to the coupling of the β-receptor and adenyl cyclase. This is the function of the Gs protein complex. It is interesting to note that 30 minutes after weaning from CPB, the β-receptor number did begin to decrease, suggesting that β-receptor downregulation may play a role in postoperative response to β-specific inotropic agents.

Schrantz and colleagues studied the effects of CPB on acyanotic pediatric patients and confirmed the experimental data obtained by Schwinn.[75] They demonstrated that after CPB, β-agonists induced increases in cyclic-AMP where attenuated. However, when several non-β-receptor-dependent stimulators of adenyl cyclase were examined, adenyl cyclase activity increased in a normal fashion despite CPB. In addition, β_1 and β_2-receptor density was found to be unaltered by CPB. These studies suggest a primary role for the Gs protein complex in the desensitization of β-agonist action during weaning from CPB period.

Pulmonary Effects

Pulmonary function after CPB is characterized by reduced static and dynamic compliance, reduced functional residual capacity, and an increased A-a gradient.[76,77] Surfactant washout, atelectasis, and increased interstitial edema and endothelial injury due to hemodilution, leukocyte aggregation, and hypothermia are the most likely etiologies.[78,79] Hemodilution reduces circulating plasma proteins, decreasing intravascular oncotic pressure, and favors water extravasation into the extravascular space. Hypothermic CPB causes endothelial injury, complement activation, and leukocyte aggregation and degranulation.[20,21,25,26] Leukocytes and complement are extremely important in promoting capillary alveolar membrane injury and microvascular dysfunction through platelet plugging and release of mediators which increase pulmonary vascular resistance and further damage to the endothelium.[80] Evidence suggests that hypothermia may be an additional factor in inducing lung injury.[17] A direct vascular endothelial injury occurs from hypothermic nonpulsatile CPB. This may be a major factor causing lung injury in addition to the endothelial effects caused by exposure of blood to the nonendothelialized bypass circuit.[17,28,30] Preliminary investigations on the effects of circulatory arrest on pulmonary function obtained from our laboratory suggests that pulmonary function deteriorates during continuous-flow CPB but does not worsen during or after the arrest period. This implies that deep hypothermic circulatory arrest may "protect" the lung from the continuous damaging effects introduced by blood exposure to the pump oxygenator.

Surfactant replacement and rapid removal of extravascular water through the technique of modified ultrafiltration have been suggested as methods for improving lung compliance and decreasing airway resistance in the immediate post-CPB period.[79] Surfactant replacement therapy improved lung compliance immediately after CPB in children undergoing ASD repair. Modified ultrafiltration, a bypass technique used to rapidly remove extravascular water from the patient immediately after weaning from CPB, has demonstrated significant and rapid improvements in lung compliance and reduction in airway resistance in preliminary data obtained at our institution.

Renal Effects

The combined effects of hypothermia, nonpulsatile perfusion, and reduced mean arterial pressure cause release of angiotensin, renin, catecholamines, and antidiuretic hormones.[27,81–83] These circulating hormones promote renal vasoconstriction, reduce total renal blood flow, and redistribute intrarenal blood flow to the renal medulla. The addition of pulsatile perfusion improves renal blood flow by inhibiting renin release and redistributing blood flow to the renal cortex.[83] Urine flow and renal tissue oxygenation are improved.[84] Yet despite the negative impact of CPB on renal function, studies have been unable to link low-flow, low-pressure, nonpulsatile perfusion with postoperative renal dysfunction.[85,86] The factor that correlates best with postoperative renal dysfunction is profound post-CPB low cardiac output and preoperative renal dysfunction. Preoperative factors include primary renal disease, low cardiac output, and dye-related renal injury after cardiac catheterization.[87,88]

Organ immaturity also results in a reduced glomerular filtration rate and medullary concentrating ability. Therefore, prolonged periods of CPB may result in greater fluid retention than is typically seen in adult patients. The net result may be increased total body water and greater difficulty with postoperative weaning from ventilatory support. The use of total circulatory arrest has been associated with postoperative acute tubular necrosis and transient elevations of blood urea nitrogen and creatinine. Using higher perfusion flow rates in the prearrest and postarrest period seems to reduce but not eliminate post-CPB renal dysfunction in patients with good postrepair myocardial function.

Cerebral Effects of Low-Flow Hypothermic CPB and Deep Hypothermic Circulatory Arrest

Although all organs are at risk for hypoxic-ischemic injury, the brain is the most sensitive and therefore the limiting factor when using low-flow CPB and DHCA. In contrast to the heart, where cardioplegic arrest has improved myocardial performance, a combination of hypothermia and nonpulsatile perfusion are the main modalities of cerebral protection currently available. For this reason we have elected to discuss hypoxic-ischemic injury from a cerebral perspective. We will discuss normothermic ischemia first and then the protective effects of hypothermia, followed by a discussion of the physiological effects of hypothermic CPB on the brain.

Ischemic Injury and Hypothermic Protection

Normothermia and Ischemic Injury. At normothermic temperatures, the energy-rich compounds (ATP and phosphocreatine) are maintained through oxidative metabolism. A majority of the ATP and phosphocreatine produced is used for maintaining ion homeostasis. In fact, it is estimated that from 50 to 75% of high-energy phosphate expenditure is for the maintenance of transmembrane ionic gradients.[89-91] Arresting the circulation at normothermia results in a rapid depletion of high-energy phosphate stores.[49] After 2 minutes of complete ischemia, ATP levels fall to 10% of prearrested values.[92] In association with ATP depletion, there is a release of excitatory neurotransmitters (i.e., glutamate, aspartate).[91-94] Neurotransmitter release is not specific to ischemia, as it can be seen with other cerebral insults, such as hypoglycemia.[95] It is believed, however, to represent a stereotypic response of ischemic injury.

Neurotransmitter release adversely affects membrane ionic permeability.[96] ATP depletion in concert with excitatory neurotransmitter release signals a dramatic alteration in the maintenance of transmembrane ionic gradients. Electrochemical gradients for potassium, calcium, and sodium are lost, presumably due to unrestricted ion permeability across cell membranes.[97] The loss of ionic gradients does not indicate a breakdown of cell membrane integrity, and although ATP levels are reduced, there is evidence to suggest that dysfunction of the energy-dependent ionic pumps does not occur within the first few minutes of normothermic ischemia.[98,99] However, low ATP levels may prevent the reestablishment of transmembrane ion gradients after the initial ion flux.

It is the influx of the ion calcium which is the harbinger of permanent cellular damage. Approximately 95% of the calcium present in the extracellular space moves into the cell during the period of increased membrane permeability.[97] Calcium influx results in accelerated cellular damage through the activation of calcium-dependent enzymes (phospholipases, nucleases, and xanthine oxidase).

Phospholipase C and A_2 release free fatty acids (FFA), such as arachidonic acid.[98] Free fatty acids are in general powerful uncouplers of oxidative phosphorylation and inhibit the exchange of adenosine diphosphate (ADP) for ATP across mitochondrial membranes. The FFA arachidonic acid is metabolized to prostaglandins through the cyclooxygenase pathway and to leukotrienes through the lipoxygenase pathway during postischemic reperfusion. Ischemia alters the composition of prostaglandin production.[98,99,100] The potent vasoconstrictors, $PGF_{2\alpha}$ and thromboxane, are produced in favor of vasodilators, such as prostacyclin (PGI_2). Thromboxane also promotes platelet aggregation resulting in small vessel thrombosis.

Leukotrienes are undetectable in the nonischemic brain.[101] However, with ischemia and reperfusion, leukotriene levels (interleukines and cytokines) increase dramatically.[102] Like prostaglandins, leukotrienes are potent cerebral vasoconstrictors. In addition, leukotrienes are mediators of "secondary ischemic damage" through increased capillary permeability and by promoting leukocyte entry into the ischemic tissue. The probable result is an amplification of FFA-mediated cell injury, permeability, cerebral edema, platelet plugging, and accelerated vascular thrombosis.

Nucleases become active after ischemia and have been implicated in creating single stranded breaks in DNA. A majority of nucleases are calcium dependent, and thus calcium entry is an important cofactor for nuclease activity.[103,104] Single-strand DNA breaks are generally easily repaired.[105] However, extensive single-stranded regions are prone to secondary breaks in the presence of oxygen-free radicals. The conversion of single-strand breaks to double-strand breaks is considered lethal to the cell.[105–108]

The enzymatic breakdown of ADP and adenosine monophosphate (AMP) not only wastes energy but also contributes to hypoxic cell damage.[107] AMP is either dephosphorylated to adenosine or deaminated to inosine monophosphate. Adenosine crosses the cell membrane through facilitated diffusion and acts as a potent local vasodilator. It is through adenosine release that the cell attempts to improve local O_2 delivery. During severe hypoxia, however, both inosine monophosphate and intracellular adenosine can be metabolized to hypothanthine. Hypothanthine in the presence of the enzyme xanthine oxidase is converted to the free radicals O_2^- and $H_2O_2^-$, which are important mediators of ischemic cerebral injury. A free radical is defined as any molecule containing an unpaired electron. In the presence of free iron, free radicals are catalyzed to potent oxidizing species which target proteins, unsaturated membrane lipids, and DNA. The result is extensive damage to cell membranes, nucleic acids, and enzyme systems.[109,110] A flow chart describing this cascade is shown in Figure 3–3.

Hypothermia and Protection from Ischemic Injury

Both the duration of the arrest period and the quality of perfusion techniques influence the development of these problems. Hypothermia seems to protect the brain from ischemic injury through preserving high-energy phosphate stores, preventing excitatory neurotransmitter release, restricting membrane permeability, and preventing calcium entry into the cell.

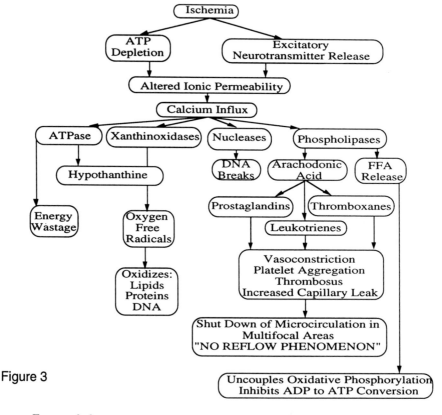

Figure 3

FIGURE 3–3. A flow chart describing the cerebral cellular events associated with normothermic arrest.

Several authors have examined the protective effect of deep hypothermia by measuring high-energy phosphate compounds with ³¹phosphate nuclear magnetic resonance (³¹P-NMR).[111–115] These authors reported that while ATP was rapidly depleted at normothermic temperatures, ATP levels were maintained at deep hypothermic temperatures (15 to 20°C) for a more prolonged period of time. At hypothermic temperatures, the rate of energy-dependent cellular enzyme systems such as, Na-K ATPase and Ca-ATPase, are drastically slowed. ATP and phosphocreatine utilization are reduced, excitatory neurotransmitter release is truncated, and ion homeostasis is maintained through both energy-dependent and -independent mechanisms. At hypothermic temperatures, ischemic events do not proceed concurrently.

Norwood and colleagues have demonstrated that 25 minutes of deep hypothermic arrest significantly lowers creatine phosphate levels, but ATP stores are well maintained in isolated perfused rat brains.[111] In contrast, larger animal studies suggest that ATP levels reach their nadir after 21 to 33 minutes of hypothermic circulatory arrest.[11,112,115] After 1 hour of circulatory arrest, ³¹P-NMR measurements suggested a delay in ATP recovery. In sheep, after 60 minutes of arrest at 15°C ATP levels were reduced to 36% of control. Thirty minutes of normothermic reperfusion, however, restored ATP levels to 83% of control values.[11] In a similar model using piglets, intracellular pH did not recover from a 60 minute arrest period until nearly 40 minutes of normothermic reperfusion. ATP and phosphocreatine levels recovered to 90 and 98% of baseline, but required 3 hours of normothermic reperfusion.[115] Studies of whole brain cerebral metabolism in both animals and children demonstrate a significant reduction after DHCA, which is not found after low-flow CPB. Therefore, both cellular levels of ATP and global measures of cerebral metabolism are both reduced after DHCA, suggesting reperfusion injury.

There are, however, discrepancies between whole brain metabolic studies and cellular ATP studies using NMR. These differences may be model dependent. The measured nadir of ATP after only 21 to 33 minutes of DHCA in large animals does not imply an absence of ATP but rather a point where ATP, ADP, and AMP levels are indistinguishable by ³¹P-NMR techniques. In addition, the loss of cellular stores of ATP does not predict the point of cellular injury. Instead it signifies the point at which the energy-dependent processes which maintain transmembrane ionic gradients is lost. Deeper levels of hypothermia as used during hypothermic CPB may prevent calcium entry through altering membrane fluidity, an energy-independent process. Additionally, alterations in cooling and reperfusion techniques may provide additional protection by ensuring more complete brain cooling prior to the arrest period or by restoring ATP levels before instituting significant cerebral rewarming, respectively.

Excitatory neurotransmitters are also mediators of ischemic injury in the brain.[116] Glutamate, for example, induces selective injury to neurons in the hippocampus.[117] Dopamine, generally regarded as an inhibitory neurotransmitter, acts as an excitatory neurotransmitter in certain brain regions, such as the D_2 receptors in the nigrostriatum.[118,119] In this region of the brain, dopamine has been implicated as a mediator of neuronal injury.

Studies of ischemic brain injury in the rat, using a four-vessel occlusion model, has demonstrated that ischemic injury results in an increased release of both glutamate and dopamine. When temperature is lowered from 36 to 33°C the expected rise in glutamate release does not occur, and dopamine levels actually fall. Interestingly, minimal levels of hypothermia (34°C) have been shown to prevent the ischemic neuronal injury on the CA-1 layer of the hippocampus when compared to normothermic controls. Moderate hypothermia of 27°C was no more protective than this slight level of hypothermia.[120,121] This suggests that excitatory neurotransmitter release may act as an accelerator of neurological injury by promoting the loss of transmembrane ionic gradients and enhancing calcium entry. More moderate levels of hypothermia may be sufficient to prevent the triggered release of excitatory neurotransmitters but do not reduce brain metabolism or alter transmembrane permeability to the same degree as more extreme hypothermic temperatures.

Deeper levels of hypothermia may provide additional protection from Ca entry through altering membrane fluidity. At deep hypothermic temperatures, it has been suggested that cellular membranes alter their permeability through changes in the physical state of membrane lipids, i.e., they become less liquid and more semisolid.[122] This may directly affect free ion movement across cellular membranes and provide additional protection once ATP-dependent mechanisms for ion homeostasis are lost.

Although deep hypothermia affords the most effective protection currently available, periods of low-flow CPB or DHCA are not without risk. Newburger and colleagues, performing sophisticated neuropsychological testing in neonates undergoing DHCA for repair of transposition of the great arteries, demonstrated a greater likelihood of developmental abnormalities and postoperative seizures in patients exposed to more prolonged periods of DHCA.[63] These data in association with previous reports suggest that DHCA should be used more judiciously; however, as we will discuss below, more efficient and rigorous cooling strategies, substitution of low-flow CPB for DHCA, reperfusion periods during the arrest period, and newer rewarming strategies may minimize the risk of DHCA and reduce neuropsychological injury.

Cerebral Effects of Hypothermic CPB

During CPB, hypothermia is the most important factor altering cerebral hemodynamic and metabolical parameters. Hypothermia produces a marked reduction in both cerebral blood flow (CBF) and brain metabolism ($CMRO_2$) at constant pump flow rates (Fig. 3–4). The coupling of flow to metabolism is an important concept in assuring adequate oxygen delivery and limiting luxuriant perfusion to the brain. Variations in flow, metabolism, and their coupling are dramatically altered by hypothermic CPB.[28,38,123]

CBF decreases in a direct linear relationship with temperature (Fig. 3–4). In studies where all of the major factors altered by the extracorporeal circulation are evaluated, i.e., CO_2, perfusion pressure, pump flow rate, and temperature, temperature is the most important factor influencing CBF during CPB in children.[28,38] Moderate and deep hypothermia have differing effects on CBF and its autoregulation.

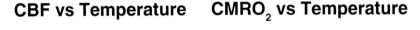

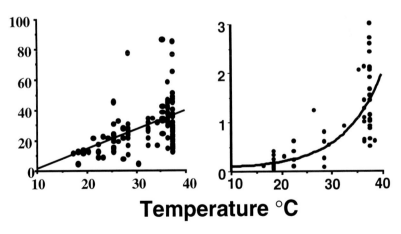

FIGURE 3–4. The effect of temperature reduction during CPB on CBF and $CMRO_2$ in children. The left side of the figure depicts the linear relationship between temperature and CBF. The right side of the figure depicts the exponential relationship between temperature and $CMRO_2$.

Pressure/flow autoregulation or the ability to maintain a constant CBF despite wide ranges in mean arterial pressures has been shown to be intact during moderate hypothermic CPB (26 to 30°C) in adults and children when measured using alpha stat blood-gas regulation.[47,123,124] The cerebral vasculature maintains a normal physiological response of dilation during low-perfusion pressure and constriction when perfusion pressure is high. In contrast, at deep hypothermic temperatures of 15 to 20°C, pressure/flow autoregulation is lost.[123] At deep hypothermic temperatures, cerebral vascular resistance (CVR) increases with temperature reduction. CVR remains high even when pump flow rates and perfusion pressure are substantially reduced.

Whereas CBF decreases in a linear fashion with reductions in brain temperature, brain metabolism ($CMRO_2$) decreases exponentially (Fig. 3–4).[38,125] A convenient expression of the effect of temperature on $CMRO_2$ is to calculate the ratio of metabolism at a temperature gradient of 10°C, called the temperature coefficient or Q_{10}.[10,126] Cerebral oxygen consumption has been measured in a number of models during CPB (dog, monkey, and man) and has been shown to vary greatly between species and at differing ages within species (Table 3–3).[38,126-128] The increased metabolical suppression for younger patients may be due to a greater susceptibility of the immature neurons and glial elements to hypothermia or may reflect greater brain mass as a percent of body weight and more efficient brain cooling. Inter- and intraspecies variability for Q_{10} may explain why variables other than temperature have been implicated as major contributors to cerebral protection during CPB. If one used adult-derived Q_{10} data, temperature-induced metabolical suppression would appear insufficient to explain clinically acceptable "safe" circulatory arrest periods, and other variables would be sought.

Because hypothermic protection alone can account for the majority of the protection seen during deep hypothermic circulatory arrest,[38] other variables, such as anesthetic agents, provide much smaller contributions to cerebral protection, once deep hypothermic temperatures (15 to 20°C) are reached.[10,127] At more moderate temperatures, anesthetic agents and other cerebroprotective agents such as calcium chan-

TABLE 3–3. Q_{10} DIFFERENCES BETWEEN SPECIES

Study	Species	Q_{10}
Michenfelder et al.[129]	Dog	2.2
Bering[130]	Monkey	3.5
Croughwell[131]	Adult human	2.8
Greeley[38]	Children	3.65

nel blockers, barbiturates, and N-methyl-D-aspartate antagonists, may be more important. If deep hypothermia is the only cerebroprotective agent employed, then factors which enhance cerebral cooling by modifying cerebral blood flow.

Cerebral blood flow decreases linearly with reductions in temperature. In contrast, cerebral metabolism decreases exponentially with reductions in temperature. Therefore, flow to metabolism ratios must increase with decreasing temperature during CPB in children. In the awake healthy child, cerebral blood flow (CBF) and metabolism ($CMRO_2$) are regulated by the metabolical needs of regional areas of the brain. This has been termed "cerebral flow/metabolism coupling" and is an important regulatory feature of cerebral homeostasis.[10,129–132] In humans, a mean CBF of 45 to 80 ml/100 gm/minute is coupled to a $CMRO_2$ of 3.0 to 4.0 ml/100 gm/minute, for a CBF to $CMRO_2$ ratio of 13 to 20/liter.[10,38,68] In neonates, $CMRO_2$, CBF, and the CBF to $CMRO_2$ ratio are generally higher than in older children and adults. This is believed to be due to increased metabolical demand for neuronal growth and myelinization, etc.[133]

If CPB is managed using alpha-stat blood gas regulation at a pump flow rate of 100 ml/kg/minute, the ratio of CBF to $CMRO_2$ increases with decreasing temperature, so that during moderate hypothermic CPB the CBF to $CMRO_2$ ratio increases to 30 to 1. At deep hypothermic temperatures the ratio of CBF to $CMRO_2$ extends to 75 to 1.[38] In contrast, pH-stat blood-gas regulation (the addition of CO_2 to the gas flow mixture) results in CBF to $CMRO_2$ ratios of 60 to 1 at moderate hypothermia.[124] Whereas at deep hypothermic temperatures flow to metabolism ratios using pH-stat strategy are unknown. Although alpha-stat regulation has been believed to maintain flow/metabolism coupling at moderate hypothermia, cerebral blood flow becomes increasingly luxuriant at lower temperatures in children even using alpha-stat blood gas regulation. Luxuriant flow becomes important when low pump flows are used in conjunction with deep hypothermic CPB.

Low-Flow CPB

Guidelines for the safe implementation of low-flow CPB are not firmly established. Recently, estimates for minimal acceptable pump flow rates (PFR) for children during CPB have been suggested. Using Q10 data, one can predict $CMRO_2$ at different temperatures. For children at 37°C, the mean $CMRO_2$ = 1.48, at 28°C mean $CMRO_2$ = 0.51 (66% reduction), at 18°C mean $CMRO_2$ = 0.16, (89% reduction), and at 15°C mean $CMRO_2$ = 0.11 (93% reduction).[38] By comparing the reduction in $CMRO_2$ with proportional reductions in pump flow rates an estimate of minimal acceptable flow rates can be predicted.[140] Both human and animal data suggest that these data represent a reasonable approximation of acceptable minimal pump flow rates during hypothermic CPB (Fig. 3–5).[11,37,47,48,50,127,128]

Deep Hypothermic Circulatory Arrest (DHCA)

Recent clinical evidence has demonstrated a higher incidence of transient postoperative seizures and psychometer dysfunction after 45 to 60 minutes of circulatory arrest when compared with low-flow continuous perfusion in neonates undergoing DHCA.[63] The implication of this new data is two-fold: 1) DHCA imparts a greater neurological risk to neonates and infants compared with continuous-flow bypass and 2) conventional methods of implementing and managing circulatory arrest does not adequately address the quality of perfusion techniques used to prepare the brain prior to DHCA initiation nor address cerebral oxygen delivery requirements immediately after a period of DHCA. Newer monitoring and protective strategies may impact significantly on postarrest neurological injury.

HCA with Intermittent Perfusion Periods

Intermittent systemic perfusion between periods of DHCA has been suggested as an alternative to prolonged periods of deep hypothermic

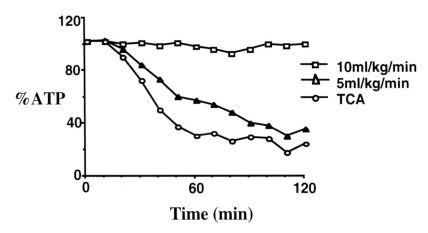

FIGURE 3–5. Comparison of the effects of low-flow CPB at either 5 ml/kg/minute or 10 ml/kg/minute with DHCA using ^{31}P-NMR. DHCA results in a marked decrease in ATP over time. Low-flow CPB at rates of 10 ml/kg/minute of flow maintains normal ATP levels, whereas 5 ml/kg/minute demonstrates a reduction in ATP levels over time which is slightly better than DHCA.

arrest. These periods of reperfusion have been suggested as a way to replete cerebral high-energy phosphate stores and preserve neurological tissue. Data investigating this concept are limited. Reperfusion periods of 1 minute at deep hypothermic temperatures between two 30-minute circulatory arrest periods significantly improved metabolical recovery when compared to a 60-minute period of circulatory arrest (Fig. 3–6).[134,135] This is consistent with NMR data, which suggest that high-energy phosphate compounds reach their nadir after approximately 30 minutes. In a sheep model, a 30-minute period of reperfusion following a 60-minute period of circulatory arrest partially restored intracellular pH, ATP, and phosphocreatine levels. A second 60-minute period of circulatory arrest, however, resulted in rapid depletion of ATP and phosphocreatine levels. After a second 60-minute period of circulatory arrest ATP, phosphocreatine, and intracellular pH values were no different than a continuous 2-hour arrest period.[11] These studies support the conclusion that 30 minutes of arrest at deep hypothermic temperatures do not result in full depletion of cellular ATP and phosphocreatine. Replenishing cellular metabolical stores may occur more rapidly at hypothermic temperatures especially if cellular levels of ATP are not fully depleted prior to reinstitution perfusion.

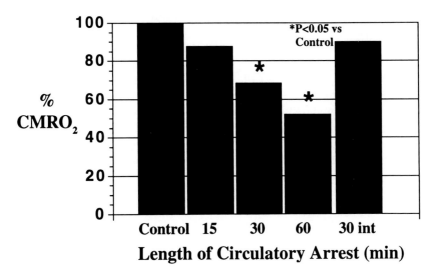

FIGURE 3–6. Percent $CMRO_2$ recovery after varying lengths of circulatory arrest in a piglet model. The longer the arrest period the less recovery of $CMRO_2$. When a 60-minute period of circulatory arrest is interrupted for 1 minute and the animal reperfused at 100 ml/kg/minute of flow, $CMRO_2$ returns to near normal levels.

Cerebral Effects of CO_2 Regulation

Elevated CO_2 tension is a potent cerebrovasodilator in both the awake and anesthetized state, with or without CPB. The addition of CO_2 by using pH-stat blood-gas regulation causes luxuriant CBF which may distribute an increased proportion of embolic material (air or particulate) to the brain rather than the systemic circulation. The concern of embolism is magnified in children for two reasons: 1) the presence of intra- and extracardiac communications between the systemic and pulmonary circulation and 2) the increased amount of intracardiac surgery performed. In addition to the risk of embolism, pH-stat strategy would increase global CBF, which may result in cerebral hyperemia and increased brain edema after prolonged periods of hemodiluted, nonpulsatile CPB.[136,137] The potential advantage of pH-stat regulation on the cerebral circulation is also luxuriant cerebral perfusion. This may be advantageous in improving brain cooling and reducing the potential hazard of cerebral steal from aortopulmonary collaterals or shunts associated with cyanotic cardiac defects. Regional areas of cerebral hypoperfusion resulting in watershed infarcts have been described in patients with shunt physiology and low diastolic blood pressure.[138]

Despite the theoretical risks associated with differing CO_2 strategies, a recent prospective study in adults comparing pH- and alpha-stat management during moderate hypothermic CPB could not demonstrate an increased neuropsychiatrical risk for either strategy (mean temperature, $30.1 \pm 2.0°C$).[139] Because CO_2 and pH effects become more important with decreasing temperature, and at low cerebral perfusion pressures CO_2 becomes less important than mean arterial pressure, the applicability of this study to children undergoing deep hypothermic CPB is limited.[126,140] At moderate hypothermic temperatures, mean differences in $PaCO_2$ between alpha-stat and pH-stat strategies at $30°C$ are between 6 and 7 mm Hg, and pH differences are approximately 0.06. In addition, at cerebral perfusion pressures of 30 mm Hg or less, CBF becomes indistinguishable from the two blood-gas management strategies. In contrast, at deep hypothermic temperatures of $17°C$, CO_2 differences may approach 80 mm Hg and pH differences 0.24.[141]

If a period of circulatory arrest is used in addition to pH-stat regulation, a further reduction in intracellular pH occurs.[37] The resultant severe cerebral acidosis may delay or prevent full brain recovery. Low pH, in addition to impairing enzymatic function, may cause iron release from transferrin. Free iron has been shown to catalyze free radical formation and result in permanent membrane damage through lipid peroxidation.[142] Therefore, intracellular acidosis during CPB with DHCA may result in greater neuronal and glial injury. pH stat worsens acidosis during and immediately after a period of DHCA.

Brain reperfusion during the rewarming period of CPB must eliminate or correct the low pH toward normal. This may be hampered by a high residual acid load after circulatory arrest and from the increasing metabolical demands of the rewarming brain. In addition, nonpulsatile perfusion may not adequately meet the metabolical demands of the brain, particularly when pH-stat blood-gas regulation is used.

Stressing the brain with a substantial metabolical debt at the end of CPB may be deleterious. Once weaned from CPB, the brain becomes dependent on the postbypass function of the heart to sustain adequate cerebral perfusion and eliminate accrued metabolical debt. If cardiac output is marginal or right atrial filling pressures high, cerebral perfusion may be inadequate for the metabolical demands of the brain tissue. Reducing acid load before separating from CPB should be beneficial.

Cerebral Cooling Strategies and DHCA

Accelerated rates of cooling ($>1°C/min$) during CPB using alpha-stat regulation are associated with a lower developmental quotient in neonates undergoing deep hypothermic circulatory arrest.[143] High cerebral oxygen extraction, low jugular venous bulb saturations, and more elevated cerebral metabolical rates than expected at 18°C suggest inadequate cerebral perfusion from inefficient brain cooling, and the existence of temperature gradients throughout the brain has been associated with neurological disability.[38] Marked variability in cerebral cooling has been established in several clinical studies. When jugular venous saturation was used as a marker for complete cerebral cooling, one-third of patients demonstrated significantly slower brain cooling.[131] When cooling techniques were varied, perfusion with colder pump blood resulted in a larger temperature gradient between the arterial blood and brain tissue and contributed to more rapid and complete cerebral cooling.[144]

Studies in the rat demonstrate temperature gradients of 2 to 6°C between deep brain structures and temporalis muscle in a study using four-vessel occlusion models of cerebral ischemia.[121,145] Significant differences in neuronal function, histopathology, free fatty acid, and excitatory neurotransmitter release were demonstrated based upon regional differences in brain temperature.[121,146,147] Animal studies also suggest that there are regional differences in the distribution of brain blood flow during hypercarbia. Deep brain structures (thalamus, brain stem, and cerebellum) receive a significantly greater percentage of cerebral blood flow than cortical structures.[147]

The ideal blood-gas management strategy for children is not categorical. Just as the surgeon must decide the appropriate temperature for hypothermic bypass and whether to use moderate flow, low flow, or circulatory arrest, the appropriateness of a blood-gas strategy depends on many modifiers. These include the degree of hypothermia, pump flow rate, use of DHCA, and cooling dynamics of the brain. Appropriate strategies can be hypothesized based on our discussion. During moderate hypothermia selecting one blood-gas management strategy over the other appears less critical, because brain intracellular pH differences are small.[139,141] During deep hypothermia with or without DHCA, the addition of CO_2 during active brain cooling could potentially improve the distribution of the cold perfusate to deep brain structures. Recent evidence suggests that pH-stat management enhances the distribution of extracorporeal perfusate to the brain and may help cool the brain more thoroughly and rapidly.[37,115,148] Although improved cooling was demonstrated in these studies, metabolical recovery after circulatory arrest was shown to be impaired, suggesting that the acid load induced by pH stat had a negative effect on enzymatic function after cerebral rewarming. To retain the benefits of pH stat on cooling and eliminate its negative effects on enzymatic function, a combined blood-gas management strategy using pH and alpha stat in succession is required. In a recently completed study, a group of animals underwent initial cooling with pH stat followed by alpha stat to eliminate residual acid load prior to the initiation of deep hypothermic circulatory arrest. This group demonstrated improved metabolical suppression over alpha stat alone and demonstrated a significant enhancement in metabolical recovery after rewarming.[148] This suggests that initial cooling with pH stat followed by alpha stat may be the best approach. A controlled clinical study evaluating this approach (combined pH- and alpha-stat cooling) is ongoing at our institution.

Other factors that may result in maldistribution of pump flow away from the cerebral circulation and contribute to inefficient cerebral cooling include: anatomical variants (large aortic to pulmonary collaterals) or technical problems (aortic and venous cannula placement).[131,149] Cyanotic patients with known aortopulmonary collaterals may benefit from the cerebrovasodilation of CO_2 during early cooling. Once cool, however, if DHCA or deep hypothermia with low flow is planned, converting to an alpha-stat strategy may help preserve intracellular brain pH and reduce postarrest cerebral acidosis.

Hypothermic Injury to the Brain

Early experience with deep hypothermia suggested that using extremely low temperatures (esophageal temperatures of less than 10°C) resulted in a dramatic increase in neurological and pulmonary injury. Neurological sequelae, especially choreoathetosis, was commonly reported.[150–152] These early reports diminished the enthusiasm for profound levels of hypothermia, and most institutions limited hypothermic temperatures to 18 to 20°C.

These early reports contrast with current practice and recent studies using more extreme levels of hypothermia. For example, a recent study supports the use of cold cerebroplegia (perfusing the brain with hemodiluted blood cooled to 6 to 10°C) as an alternative to hypothermic arrest during aortic arch surgery in adults.[153] This group reports reduced neurological injury using this technique.

Current practice at many pediatric cardiac centers is to use a water bath temperature of 4°C and cool rapidly until the rectal temperature reaches 15°C. Using this technique it is not uncommon to reach esophageal temperatures below 10°C and tympanic membrane temperatures of between 10 and 12°C. This cooling strategy has not resulted in a clinically demonstrable increased incidence of neurological sequelae when compared to more traditional cooling techniques, although controlled clinical comparative trials have not been documented.

The difference between earlier studies and current experience is most likely due to hemodilution. All of the early reports used surface cooling techniques and did not hemodilute. At low temperatures the viscosity of blood increases, red cell deformity is reduced, and microvascular sludging results. The brain becomes hypoperfused in multifocal areas (the pathological picture of no reflow), and brain injury results. The use of deep hypothermia with hemodilution eliminates these no-reflow lesions.[49] However, hypothermia does result in alterations in microvascular function (endothelial injury), as discussed previously.

The limit at which hypothermia causes significant end-organ damage is not known. Current clinical practice suggests, however, that temperatures of 15°C and below are probably no worse than temperatures of 18 to 20°C, as long as appropriate hemodilution is used.

THE PEDIATRIC EXTRACORPOREAL CIRCUIT

The trend in modern pediatric bypass equipment is to reduce the size of the extracorporeal circuit in order to reduce the prime volume. Current circuit designs require a very large priming volume when compared to the blood volume of neonates and small infants. The priming volume may actually exceed the blood volume of a neonate by as much as 200 to 300%. This is in contrast to an adult CPB patient where the priming volume accounts for only 25 to 33% of the patient's blood volume.

The larger priming volumes required for neonates and infants have two pronounced disadvantages: 1) donor blood must be added to the prime and 2) marked hemodilution occurs after initiation of CPB. The use of donor blood has several disadvantages, including viral transmission, complement activation, and high levels of glucose and lactate transfused into infants along with citrate-phosphate-dextrose (CPD) stored blood.[154,155] Hemodilution during CPB results in reductions in plasma proteins and clotting factors, decreased colloid osmotic pressure, resulting in enhanced interstitial edema, electrolyte imbalance, and an exaggerated release of stress hormones, complement, and white blood cell and platelet activation. For these reasons, manufacturers are finding themselves under increasing scrutiny to develop miniaturized components that lessen the effect of the priming volume on the pediatric patient. Until then, care must be taken to achieve a physiologically balanced prime and to anticipate the potential impact of transfusion and marked hemodilution on the pediatric CPB patient.

Hemodilution is necessitated during hypothermic CPB, because blood viscosity increases as temperature is lowered. Hematocrits of 40% coupled with hypothermia and the nonpulsatile flow of CPB impair blood flow through the microcirculation. Blood sludging with small vessel occlusion and multiple areas of cerebral hypoperfusion have been described in experimental models.[49,156,157]

Defining the optimal level of hemodilution during pediatric CPB is based on assuring adequate oxygen delivery at hypothermic temperatures and during rewarming. Hematocrits as low as 10% appear to provide adequate oxygen delivery during hypothermic CPB based on animal studies and observations in patients who are Jehovah's Witnesses.[158,159] The safety, however, of hematocrits below 15% has been questioned because of the difficulty of assuring adequate oxygen delivery during the rewarming period.[160]

Oxygenators

In the pediatric population, oxygenators must provide efficient gas exchange over a wide range of temperatures (10 to 40°C), pump flow rates (0 to 200 ml/kg/min), hematocrit (15 to 30%), line pressures, and gas flow rates. Both bubble and membrane oxygenators can achieve effective gas exchange under these diverse conditions. Bubble oxygenators allow fresh gas, in the form of microbubbles, to mix directly with circulating blood in an oxygenating column. The direct interface of blood and gas is traumatic to blood cellular elements, causing increased red blood cell hemolysis, platelet microaggregation, complement activation, and release of mediators of the inflammatory response.[14,29–31,60] These undesirable effects are minimized with the use of membrane oxygenators.

The membrane oxygenator acts as a synthetic alveolar-capillary membrane, where a direct interface between the blood and fresh gas is minimized or absent. Most membrane oxygenators used for CPB are composed of microporous hollow fibers. A microporous membrane contains pores of 3 to 5 μm in size which allow a minimal contact between the blood and gas. The advantage of micropores is improved gas exchange with a smaller total membrane surface area. The disadvantage is that if negative pressure develops on the blood side of the membrane, gas emboli can be entrained into the blood and result in gas embolization in the arterial blood of the patient.

A third type of membrane oxygenator is composed of nonporous silicone and is arranged in folded sheets. Nonporous silicone membrane oxygenators are more expensive and require a larger surface area for gas exchange than microporous membranes. Silicone membranes provide no clear advantage for short-term perfusion but are the only membrane oxygenator recommended for long-term perfusion such as extracorporeal membrane oxygenation (ECMO) support.

Pumps

There are two types of pumps currently used for CPB: roller pumps and centrifugal pumps. Roller pumps are the most widely used in pediatric perfusion. Roller pumps consist of two rollers which are oriented 180° from each other. They provide continuous blood flow by partially occluding the tubing between the roller and the pump casing. Blood is displaced in a forward direction by the roller causing continuous, nonpulsatile flow. The second roller acts as a valve to minimize back flow. The rollers are never totally occlusive because that would encourage hemolysis. Maladjustment in occlusion can result in a higher percentage error in estimating pump flow rate and increased red cell hemolysis.

Centrifugal pumps are newer devices, which are of increasing interest because of experience gained in ECMO and ventricular assist devices. Flow is maintained by the entrainment of blood against spinning impellers (curved blades) or by creating a vortex utilizing a centrifugal cone. The advantages of centrifugal pumps are: a reduced priming volume, less damage to formed blood elements, and the vortex design which may assist in air removal.[162] These pumps are also capable of producing pulsatile blood flow which may improve flow in the microcirculation. An example is the Biomedicus pump.

Tubing

Tubing size should be kept as small as possible to reduce prime volume but must be large enough to achieve effective flow rates and low line pressure. Both the length and the diameter of the tubing contributes to prime volume. In neonates, quarter inch tubing is used for both the arterial and venous limbs of the circuit. Tube length is kept as short as possible by positioning the pump close to the surgical field. Quarter-inch tubing requires approximately 30 ml of volume per meter of tube length.

Cardiotomy Circuit

The cardiotomy circuit is used to suction blood from the field and return it to the patient's circulation. It requires its own reservoir, roller pump, and filters. Suction tubing from the cardiotomy circuit can be attached to free suckers in the operative field or to aortic, atrial, or ventricular vents. Once collected, the blood is drained into a venous reservoir which can then be added to the venous inflow of the oxygenator. These open systems with large reservoirs require complete or full heparinization to prevent clot formation in the stagnant blood contained in the reservoir. ECMO which is a closed system without a reservoir requires less heparinization (ACTs of 160 to 200) to inhibit blood coagulation. Closed systems require a lesser prime but have not gained acceptance in this country due to the difficulty in administering volume in rapid fashion.

Cannulas

In neonates and infants, the cannula tip must be small to facilitate insertion into tiny aortas, while not impeding the normal flow of aortic blood around the cannula. Maintaining flow around the cannula is particularly important prior to initiating CPB and after weaning from

CPB when the cannula can significantly impede aortic outflow in small infants. Adequate perfusion flow rates must be attainable at relatively low perfusion pressures. Excessive pressure in the cannula tip may create a powerful jet of blood which could damage the intima of the aorta and blood cellular elements.

Arterial Cannulation

The arterial cannula is generally placed into the ascending aorta; however, the child's great vessel anatomy and the type of surgical procedure may influence arterial cannula placement. For example, in hypoplastic left heart syndrome the ascending aorta is 1 to 5 mm in size, too small to accept a cannula capable of providing systemic perfusion. As an alternative, the arterial cannula is placed in the main pulmonary artery. Systemic perfusion is maintained from the pulmonary artery through the ductus arteriosus and down the descending aorta. Coronary perfusion is retrograde through the hypoplastic ascending aorta. In newborns with transposition of the great arteries, the arterial cannula is placed in a more distal aspect of the ascending aorta, because a large portion of the surgery occurs on the aortic root. Infants with interrupted aortic arch require two aortic cannulas: one in the ascending aorta to perfuse the head vessels and one in the descending aorta to perfuse the body. Arterial cannulation of the femoral artery is not commonly used in neonatal or infant heart surgery because the femoral vessels are too small. In older children requiring reoperation, sternotomy may pose a high risk of inadvertently entering a conduit or a ventricular chamber. In these patients femoral cannulation should be considered.

Problems with aortic cannula placement are possible in neonates and infants. The tip of the aortic cannula may be beyond the takeoff of the innominate artery and, therefore, flow to the right side of the cerebral circulation may be retrograde through the circle of Willis. Similarly, the position of the aortic cannula may promote preferential flow down the aorta or induce a Venturi effect to steal flow from the cerebral circulation. This problem has been suggested during xenon CBF monitoring by noting large discrepancies in CBF between the right and left hemisphere after initiating CPB.[131] Placement of the aortic cannula in a more distal location, commonly employed in procedures where ascending aorta or proximal aortic arch reconstruction is required (arterial switch procedure), may play a role in altering brain blood flow. We have observed that cooling patterns are substantially different in neonates and infants compared to what is commonly observed in the adult or older child.[131] We frequently observe rectal cooling preceding tympanic membrane or nasopharyngeal cooling. This pattern suggests that a disproportionate amount of pump flow may be directed away from the cerebral circulation and may contribute to inefficient brain cooling.

Venous Cannulation

Venous anatomy can be very complex. Bilateral superior vena cava (SVC), inferior vena cava (IVC) which drain into an azygous vein or hemiazygous vein, or hepatic veins which drain directly into an atrial chamber are common anatomical variations occurring in the venous system of congenital cardiac patients. Venous cannulation must account for these variables if the repair is to take place during continuous flow CPB.

If the repair is going to take place under deep hypothermic circulatory arrest, CPB is used as a cooling vehicle. The repair occurs during the arrest period. Venous cannulation can therefore be simplified. A large single venous cannula is placed in the right atrium to achieve effective venous drainage. Once cooled, the cannulas are removed and surgery proceeds in a cannula-free field. In contrast, repairs performed during continuous flow must address the complex venous anatomy. This is particularly true in single ventricle patients where left-sided SVCs are commonly found.

In the modified Fontan operation, for example (a total cavopulmonary anastomosis for patients with a single ventricle), as many as three venous cannulas may be required. A venous cannula must be placed at the SVC/innominate junction, inasmuch as the operation requires a direct anastomosis of the SVC to the right pulmonary artery. The IVC is cannulated with a short, straight cannula and is inserted below the pericardial reflection. A short cannula avoids placing the cannula tip beyond the hepatic veins and causing hepatic venous obstruction. A third venous cannula may be required if a large left SVC is present.

Appropriate placement of venous cannulas is important in achieving effective systemic perfusion. A malpositioned venous cannula has the potential for vena caval obstruction. The problems of venous obstruction are magnified during CPB because of low perfusion pressures. This is particularly true in the neonate. The use of large relatively stiff venous cannulas easily distort these very pliable great veins.

A cannula in the IVC may obstruct venous return from the splanchnic bed resulting in ascites from increased hydrostatic pressure and/or directly reduce perfusion pressure across the mesenteric, renal, and hepatic vascular beds. Significant renal, hepatic, and gastrointestinal dysfunction may ensue and should be anticipated in the patient with unexplained ascites after weaning from CPB. Similar cannulation problems may result in SVC obstruction. This problem may result in elevated jugular venous pressure, decreased cerebral perfusion pressure, and cerebral edema. Observations of reduced cerebral blood flow velocity, using transcranial Doppler monitoring, during transient occlusion of the SVC cannula have been made (personal observation). In the operating room we advise monitoring the SVC pressures directly via an internal jugular line or by looking at the patient's head for signs of increased puffiness or venous distention after initiating bypass. Discussions with the perfusionist regarding adequacy of venous return should alert the anesthesiologist and the surgeon to potential venous cannula problems. Patients with anomalies of the large systemic veins, i.e., persistent left SVC or azygous continuation of an interrupted IVC, are at particular risk for venous cannulation problems.[13]

Initiation of CPB

Once the aortic and venous cannulas are positioned and connected to the arterial and venous limb of the extracorporeal circuit, bypass is initiated. The technique for initiating bypass varies, depending on the size of the patient and the temperature of the perfusate.

In older children and adolescents, bypass is initiated slowly. The venous line is unclamped, and blood is siphoned from the right atrium into the oxygenator by gravity drainage. The rate at which venous blood is drained from the patient is determined by the height difference between the patient and the oxygenator inlet and the diameter of the venous cannula and line tubing. Venous drainage can be enhanced by increasing the height difference between the oxygenator and the patient. It can be reduced by either decreasing the height difference between the oxygenator and the patient or by partially clamping the venous line.

Once venous blood begins to accumulate in the oxygenator, the arterial pump is slowly started. Its speed is gradually increased until full flow is reached. If return is diminished, line pressure is high, or mean arterial pressure excessive, pump flow rates must be reduced. High line pressure and inadequate venous return are usually due to malposition or kinking of the arterial and venous cannulas, respectively.

In neonates and infants deep hypothermia is commonly used. For this reason, the pump prime is usually cold (18 to 22°C). When the cold perfusate contacts the myocardium, heart rate immediately slows and contraction is severely impaired. The contribution to total blood flow pumped by the heart rapidly diminishes. Therefore, to sustain adequate systemic perfusion at or near normothermic temperatures, the arterial pump must reach full flows quickly. A major difference in the initiation of bypass in neonates and infants vs older children is the speed in which full support must be achieved. One method for initiating CPB in infants is to begin the arterial pump first; once the aortic flow is assured, the venous line is unclamped, and blood is siphoned out of the right atrium into the inlet of the oxygenator. Flowing before unclamping the venous line prevents the potential problem of patient exsanguination if aortic dissection or malplacement of the aortic cannula has occurred. Pump flow rates are then rapidly increased to sustain systemic perfusion. Because coronary artery disease is not a consideration, the myocardium should cool evenly. When a cold prime is used caution must be exercised in using the pump to infuse volume prior to initiating CPB. Infusion of cold perfusate may result in bradycardia and impaired cardiac contractility before the surgeon is prepared to initiate CPB.

Once CPB begins, it is essential to observe the heart. Ineffective venous drainage can rapidly result in ventricular distention. This is especially true in infants and neonates where ventricular compliance is low and the heart is relatively intolerant of excessive preload augmentation due to a flat Starling curve.[163] If distention occurs, pump flow must be reduced and the venous cannula repositioned. Alternatively, the heart may be vented or a pump sucker placed into the right atrium.

WEANING FROM CPB

When weaning from CPB the heart is allowed to fill by partially clamping the venous return line and reducing the arterial inflow until adequate blood volume is achieved. Blood volume is assessed by direct visualization of the heart and measuring right atrial or left atrial filling pressures. When filling pressures are adequate the venous cannula is clamped, and the arterial inflow is stopped. The arterial cannula is left in place so that a slow infusion of residual pump blood can be used to optimize filling pressures. Myocardial function is assessed by direct cardiac visualization, intracardiac monitoring, and intraoperative echocardiography. In corrected physiology the pulse oximeter can also be used as a crude measure of cardiac output.[164] Low saturations or the inability of the oximeter probe to register a pulse may be a sign of very low output and high systemic resistance.[165]

After the repair of complex congenital heart defects the anesthesiologist and surgeon may have difficulty weaning patients from CPB. Under these circumstances a distinction must be made among 1) a poor surgical result with a residual defect requiring rerepair, 2) pulmonary artery hypertension, and 3) right or left ventricular dysfunction. Two methods of evaluation are used in the operating room. An intraoperative "cardiac catheterization" is performed to assess isolated pressure measurements from the various chambers of the heart, catheter pull-back measurements to evaluate residual pressure gradients across valves, repaired sites of stenosis, and conduits, and oxygen saturation data to look for residual shunts.[166] In addition, intraoperative echocardiography with Doppler color flow has been used to provide an intraoperative "picture" of structural or functional abnormalities to assist in the evaluation of the postoperative cardiac repair and ventricular function.[167] If structural abnormalities are found, the patient can be placed back on CPB, and residual defects can be repaired prior to leaving the operating room. Leaving the operating room with a significant residual structural defect adversely affects survival and increases patient morbidity.[167–170]

Functional problems are also identified by echocardiography. Once diagnosed, therapy can be directed to the specific problem. Left ventricular dysfunction can be treated by optimizing preload and heart rate, increasing coronary perfusion pressure, correcting ionized calcium levels, and adding inotropic support. Uncoupling of the β-receptor from cyclic AMP occurs during CPB, and this has been suggested as a major contributing factor for failure of beta-specific inotropic support immediately after CPB.[74,75] Inotropic support is usually begun with calcium supplementation (10 mg/kg) and dopamine (5 to 15 μg/kg/min). If function remains poor a second drug is usually added. For left ventricular dysfunction, a more potent inotrope is generally begun, such as epinephrine at a dose of 0.05 to 0.1 μg/kg/minute and titrated to effect. Dobutamine may be used as an alternative second line drug. However, due to its weak β-agonist effect, and the uncoupling of the β-receptor during CPB discussed above, it may not be efficacious to use beta-specific drugs, such as dobutamine, when weaning from CPB. In addition, dobutamine in conjunction with dopamine may produce significant tachycardia in neonates and infants. This may relate to structural similarities between dobutamine and isoproterenol.[171,172] Amrinone in conjunction with epinephrine has been shown to improve left ventricular contractility and reduce systemic afterload.[173,174] This combination is very effective for left ventricular dysfunction because it addresses left ventricular contractility through non-β-receptor-mediated mechanisms (epinephrine-α-receptor, amrinone-phosphodoesterase inhibition), an important approach after pediatric CPB. If very high doses of inotrope are required to wean from CPB, consideration for mechanical circulatory support with ECMO or a left ventricular assist device (LVAD) should be considered.

Pulmonary artery hypertension is a common problem after hypothermic CPB in children. It is best treated with alkalinization oxygen supplementation and by maintaining function residual capacity (FRC). The goal is to reduce pulmonary vascular resistance by regulating $Paco_2$, pH, PAO_2 (alveolar), PaO_2 (arterial), and FRC. Arterial pH is a potent mediator of pulmonary vascular resistance (PVR) especially in the newborn.[175] Maintaining a pH of 7.50 to 7.60 by manipulating $Paco_2$ or pH is effective in modulating PVR.[176,177] Both the arteriolar (PaO_2) and the alveolar (PAO_2) partial pressure of oxygen decrease PVR.[178] Since increasing FiO_2 reduces PVR in patients with intracardiac shunts, one can infer a direct pulmonary vasodilatory effect of the alveolar rather than arterial Po_2.

Maintaining FRC through ventilatory mechanics also plays a major role in controlling pulmonary vascular resistance. After CPB, total lung water is increased, lung compliance is reduced, and closing capacity exceeds functional residual capacity. Airway closure occurs prior to end exhalation, producing areas of lung which are perfused yet underventilated.[179,180] These segments of lung become increasingly hypoxemic, and secondary hypoxic vasoconstriction occurs. The result is elevated PVR and reduced pulmonary blood flow. When one examines set tidal volume (recorded at the ventilator) and delivered tidal volume (measured at the endotracheal tube), a large discrepancy is found. Maintaining lung volumes by using large set tidal volumes will maintain lung volumes, restore FRC, and decrease PVR.[181] Therefore, not only is hyperventilation and alkalosis important, but achieving and maintaining lung volumes are crucial. Care, however, must be taken to avoid excessive positive end-expiratory pressure or high mean airway pressure, as this may result in alveolar overdistention, compression of capillaries in the alveolar wall and interstitium, elevated PVR, reduced pulmonary blood flow, and decreased left ventricular filling.[182] Therefore, high tidal volume ventilation with I:E ratios of 1:3 or longer may be necessary to optimize lung volumes and reduce PVR when weaning from CPB.

High-frequency jet ventilation (HFJV) provides improved CO_2 removal at lower mean airway pressures. Because HFJV reduces mean airway pressure and pulmonary vascular resistance it should be ideally suited for patients with right ventricular dysfunction as well as patients with pulmonary artery hypertension. This technique is discussed in the postoperative care section.

Nitric oxide (NO) is an endothelium-derived vasodilator which can be administered as an inhaled gas. Although a nonselective smooth muscle vasodilator, NO is rapidly inactivated by hemoglobin, and therefore when administered via an inhaled route, the systemic circulation is protected from its vasodilating properties. Reduction in pulmonary vascular resistance has been demonstrated in adult patients with mitral valve stenosis and recently in children with reactive pulmonary hypertension after congenital heart surgery.[184-186] Experience with NO in the operating room has been limited.

More traditional drug therapy for elevations in pulmonary vascular resistance is of limited benefit. Phophodiesterase inhibitors, isoproterenol, prostaglandin E$_1$ (PGE$_1$), and tolazoline are not selective pulmonary vasodilators. Phophodiesterase inhibitors reduce pulmonary vascular resistance and may increase right ventricular contractility. Myocardial oxygen consumption is not significantly increased, and heart rate is not elevated.[187-190] Isoproterenol increases myocardial oxygen consumption, increases heart rate, and reduces systemic arterial pressure, all three of which may reduce coronary perfusion and contribute to right ventricular ischemia.[191,192] This is especially true if pulmonary pressures remain high and right ventricular subendocardial perfusion is impaired. PGE$_1$ and prostacyclin have been used to treat pulmonary hypertensive crises with varying degrees of success.[193] Reports of hypotension due to systemic vasodilation with both drugs has limited their use for post-CPB therapy.[175]

Right ventricular dysfunction can be treated with inotropes, by transiently increasing coronary perfusion pressure with Neo-Synephrine or epinephrine and by reducing pulmonary artery pressure to unload the right ventricle as discussed above.[174,194] It is important to remember that the right ventricle is dependent on systolic as well as diastolic pressure for coronary perfusion.[195] Therefore, drug therapy must maintain systemic perfusion pressure. PGE$_1$ or tolazoline, for example, may result in substantial systemic hypotension and be counterproductive.[193] If right ventricular dysfunction and pulmonary artery hypertension persist, cardiac output can be augmented through creating a small ASD or leaving a residual persistant foramen ovale to allow blood to shunt at the atrial level. This approach improves left ventricular filling, augments cardiac output, and improves oxygen delivery to tissue. Finally, leaving the chest open allows the right ventricle to obtain a larger end-diastolic dimension, thereby improving diastolic filling and right ventricular stroke volume. This may be necessary in neonates and infants with right heart dysfunction after weaning from CPB. If these methods fail, consideration for mechanical circulatory support should be considered.

Mechanical Circulatory Assistance in Pediatric Patients

Mechanical circulatory assistance for the failing heart is achieving wide application in adult cardiac patients. Three modalities are currently available for circulatory support in children. These include the intraaortic balloon pump (IABP), extracorporeal membrane oxygenation (ECMO), and ventricular assist devices (VADs). The need for mechanical circulatory support in the congenital heart patient is demonstrated by: 1) inability to wean from CPB due to primary ventricular dysfunction, i.e., correctable residual anatomical defects have been eliminated, 2) failure of selective surgical interventions used to reduce volume or pressure load on an unaccepting ventricle, i.e., placing a small hole in an ASD patch to allow a dysfunctional right ventricle to shunt blood right to left at the atrial level and reduce its volume load, 3) successful weaning from bypass but escalating inotropic support due to an evolving picture of ventricular dysfunction, and 4) severe pulmonary artery hypertension despite maximal ventilatory support, systemic alkalization, and inotropic support.

It is important to emphasize that care must be taken to assure that the problem is functional and not anatomical. Inotropic and ventricular assistance cannot overcome a poor operative result.[167,168,196] Intraoperative echo studies have shown an enhanced mortality if the patient leaves the operating room with a residual anatomical defect. Echocardiography and/or pressure monitoring may be used to localize the ventricular dysfunction to a right, left, or biventricular problem and eliminate residual VSDs, ASDs, and outflow or conduit obstruction. Once anatomical defects are eliminated and functional problems identified, mechanical circulatory assistance can be considered.

Modified Ultrafiltration

A modified form of ultrafiltration (MUF) which is initiated and completed within the first 15 to 20 minutes after cessation of bypass has been proposed as an effective method of decreasing total body water, reducing blood transfusion requirements, improving post-CPB hemodynamics and lung compliance after congenital cardiac surgery.[197,198] MUF uses the roller pump to pump blood through an ultrafiltration filter. Using this technique, the pump and patient hematocrit can be raised from 18 to 20 to the high 40s in minutes. The average volume of filtrate removed from the patient-pump system in a neonate is 500 to 750 ml. Although this is a new approach to post-CPB management, there are several features of modified ultrafiltration that are attractive in the immediate weaning from CPB and that may improve post-CPB end-organ function. These include: 1) lowering total body water and improving pulmonary function; 2) removing cytokines and complement from the circulation which may result in myocardial depression; 3) hemoconcentrate the circulating blood volume (including red blood cells, coagulation factors, and platelets); and

4) increasing oxygen delivery through an acute increase in circulating red blood cells which would theoretically improve oxygen delivery to the myocardium and improve myocardial contractility and cardiac output. Naik and colleagues demonstrated elevated levels of vasopeptides and interleukins in the ultrafiltrate and suggest that these may contribute to decreased myocardial function after CPB.[197,198] Preliminary work from our group suggests a significant increase in pulmonary compliance, a reduction in airway resistance, and an increase in cerebral oxygen delivery and metabolism after CPB and DHCA. More and more centers are using this technique and preliminary data derived from pediatric patients treated with modified ultrafiltration suggest a potentially important role for this technique after CPB. This subject is discussed in more depth in this monograph.

CONCLUSION

Extracorporeal circulation has evolved into a safe and effective means of circulatory support for children requiring cardiac surgery. The patient's size and age are no longer limiting factors preventing early surgical intervention and intracardiac repair. Mortality rates have fallen, especially in neonatal operation, as improvements in technology and anesthesia care have made CPB safer for neonates, infants, and children. Yet, despite the improvements, extracorporeal circulation's impact on normal physiology remains extreme. High pump-priming volumes, hypothermic temperatures, hemodilution, an exaggerated stress response, direct end-organ injury, and the use of low-flow hypothermic CPB and DHCA are problems either directly related to extracorporeal circulation or are necessitated by limits of our current technology. In the next decade, improvements in extracorporeal technology, organ protection, and managing the stress response should improve the safety of extracorporeal circulation in children and reduce post-CPB morbidity.

References

1. Blalock A, Taussig HB: The surgical treatment of malformations of the heart in which there is pulmonary stenosis or pulmonary atresia. JAMA 128:189–202, 1945
2. Potts WJ, Smith S, Gibson S: Anastamosis of the aorta to a pulmonary artery. JAMA (132):627–632, 1946
3. Bigelow WG, Lindsay WK, Greenwood WF: An investigation of factors governing survival in dogs at low body temperature. Ann Surg 132: 849–850, 1950

4. Bigelow WG, Callaghan JC, Hoppes JA: General hypothermia for experimental intracardiac surgery. Ann Surg 132:531–534, 1950
5. Borema I, Wildschut A, Schmidt WJH et al: Experimental researches into hypothermia as an aid in the surgery of the heart. Arch Chir Neerl 3: 25–30, 1951
6. Gibbon JH: Application of a mechanical heart and lung apparatus to cardiac surgery. Minnesota Med 37:171–177, 1954
7. Lillehei CW, Varco RL, Cohen M et al: The first open-heart repairs of ventricular septal defect, atrioventricularis communis, and tetralogy of Fallot using extracorporeal circulation by cross-circulation: A 30-year follow-up. Ann Thorac Surg 41:4–21, 1986
8. Warden HE: C. Walton Lillehei: Pioneer cardiac surgeon. J Thorac Cardiovasc Surg 98:833–845, 1989
9. Kirklin JW: The middle 1950's and C. Walton Lillehei. J Thorac Cardiovasc Surg 98:822–824, 1986
10. Michenfelder JD: The hypothermic brain. In Michenfelder JD (ed): Anesthesia and the Brain, pp. 23–34. New York, Churchill Livingstone, 1988
11. Swain JA, McDonald TJ, Griffith PK et al: Low flow hypothermic cardiopulmonary bypass protects the brain. J Thorac Cardiovasc Surg 102: 76–84, 1991
12. Fox LS, Blackstone EH, Kirklin JW et al: Relationship of whole body oxygen consumption to perfusion flow rate during hypothermic cardiopulmonary bypass. J Thorac Cardiovasc Surg 83:239–248, 1982
13. Hickey PR, Wessel DL (eds): Anesthesia for treatment of congenital heart disease. In Kaplan JA (ed): Cardiac Anesthesia, 2nd ed., vol. 2, pp. 635–723. Philadelphia, WB Saunders, 1987
14. Hindmarsh KW, Sankaran K, Watson VG: Plasma beta-endorphin concentrations in neonates associated with acute stress. Dev Pharmacol Ther 7:198, 1984
15. Greeley WJ, Leslie JB, Su M: Plasma atrial naturetic peptide release during pediatric cardiovascular anesthesia and surgery. Anesthesiology 65(A414):1986, 1986
16. Anand KJS, Hansen DD, Hickey PR: Hormonal-metabolic stress response in neonates undergoing cardiac surgery. Anesthesiology 73(4):661, 1990
17. Bui KC, Hammerman C, Hirshl RB et al: Plasma prostanoids in neonates with pulmonary hypertension treated with conventional therapy and with extracorporeal membrane oxygenation. J Thorac Cardiovasc Surg 101:973–983, 1991
18. Anand KJS, Sippell WG, Aynsley-Green A: Randomized trial of fentanyl anesthesia in preterm neonates undergoing surgery: Effects on the stress response. Lancet 1:243, 1987
19. Langercrantz H, Slotkin TA: The "stress" of being born. Sci Am 1: 100–107, 1986
20. Downing SW, Edmonds LH: Release of vasoactive substances during cardiopulmonary bypass. Ann Thorac Surg 54:1236–1243, 1992
21. Butler J, Rocker GM, Westaby S: Inflammatory responses to cardiopulmonary bypass. Ann Thorac Surg 55:552–559, 1993
22. Kirklin JK, Westaby S, Blackstone EH: Complement and the damaging effects of cardiopulmonary bypass. J Thorac Cardiovasc Surg 86:845–857, 1983
23. Steinberg JB, Kapelanski DP, Olson JD et al: Cytokine and complement levels in patients undergoing cardiopulmonary bypass. J Thorac Cardiovasc Surg 106:1008–1016, 1993

24. Cave AC, Manache A, Derias NW et al: Tromboxane A2 mediates pulmonary hypertension after cardiopulmonary bypass in the rabbit. J Thorac Cardiovasc Surg 106:959–967, 1993
25. Finn A, Dreyer WJ: Neutrophil adhesion and the inflammatory response induced by cardiopulmonary bypass. Cardiol Young 3:244–250, 1993
26. Howard RJ, Crain C, Franzini DA et al: Effects of cardiopulmonary bypass on pulmonary leukostasis and complement activation. Arch Surg 123:1496–1501, 1988
27. Watkins L Jr, Lucas SK, Gardner TJ et al: Angiotensin II levels during cardiopulmonary bypass: A comparison of pulsatile and nonpulsatile flow. Surg Forum 29:229–235, 1978
28. Greeley WJ, Bushman GA, Kong DL et al: Effects of cardiopulmonary bypass on ecosanoid metabolism during pediatric cardiovascular surgery. J Thorac Cardiovasc Surg 95:842–849, 1988
29. Ylikorkala O, Saarela E, Viinikka L: Increased prostacyclin and thromboxane production in man during cardiopulmonary bypass. J Thorac Cardiovasc Surg 82:245–247, 1981
30. Faymonville ME, Derby-Dupont G, Larbuisson R et al: Prostaglandin E2, prostacyclin and thromboxane changes during nonpulsatile cardiopulmonary bypass in humans. J Thorac Cardiovasc Surg 91:858–866, 1986
31. Zapol WM, Peterson MB, Wonders TR et al: Plasma thromboxane and prostacyclin metabolites in sheep partial cardiopulmonary bypass. Trans Am Soc Artif Intern Organs 26:556–560, 1980
32. Chiba Y, Muraoka R, Ihaya A et al: The effects of leukocyte depletion on the prevention of reperfusion injury during cardiopulmonary bypass. J Thorac Cardiovasc Surg 1993
33. Kelm M, Feelisch M, Deussen A et al: Release of endothelium derived nitric oxide in relation to pressure and flow. Cardiovasc Res 25:831–836, 1991
34. Ogata T, Ida Y, Nonoyama A et al: A comparative study of the effectiveness of pulsatile and nonpulsatile flow in extracorporeal circulation. Arch Jpn Clin 29:59, 1960
35. Matsumato T, Wolferth CC Jr, Perlman MH: Effects of pulsatile and nonpulsatile perfusion upon cerebral and conjunctival microcirculation in the dog. Am Surg 37:61–64, 1971
36. Geha AS, Salayemeh MT, Abe T et al: Effect of pulsatile cardiopulmonary bypass on cerebral metabolism. J Surg Res 12:381–387, 1972
37. Watanabe T, Hrita H, Kobayashi M et al: Brain tissue pH, oxygen tension and carbon dioxide tension in profoundly hypothermic cardiopulmonary bypass. J Thorac Cardiovasc Surg 97(3):396–401, 1989
38. Greeley WJ, Kern FH, Ungerleider RM et al: The effect of hypothermic cardiopulmonary bypass and total circulatory arrest on cerebral metabolism in neonates, infants and children. J Thorac Cardiovasc Surg 101:783–794, 1991
39. Davies PF, Tripathi SC: Mechanical stress mechanisms and the cell: An endothelial paradigm. Circ Res 72:239–245, 1993
40. Lefer AM, Tsao PS, Lefer DJ et al: Role of endothelial dysfunction in the pathogenesis of reperfusion injury after myocardial ischemia. FASEB J 5:2029–2034, 1991
41. Murkin JM, Farrar JK: The influence of pulsatile vs non-pulsatile bypass on cerebral blood flow and cerebral metabolism. Anesthesiology 71:A41, 1989

42. Louagi YA, Gonzalez M, Collard E et al: Does flow character of cardiopulmonary bypass make a difference? J Thorac Cardiovasc Surg 104: 1628–1634, 1992

43. Vigneswaran WT, Pollock JES, Jamieson, MPG et al: Plasma levels of glucose, insulin, and cortisol in children undergoing cardiac surgery: Effects of pulsatile and nonpulsatile perfusion. Perfusion 4:33–40, 1989

44. Lazenby WD, Ko W, Zelano JA et al: Effects of temperature and flow rate on regional blood flow and metabolism during cardiopulmonary bypass. Ann Thorac Surg 54:449–459, 1981

45. Sabiston DC Jr, Theilen EO, Gregg DE: The relationship of coronary blood flow and cardiac output and other parameters in hypothermia. Surgery 38:498–505, 1955

46. Mavroudis C, Brown GL, Katzmark SL et al: Blood flow distribution on infant pigs subjected to surface cooling, deep hypothermia, and circulatory arrest. J Thorac Cardiovasc Surg 87:665–672, 1984

47. Govier AV, Reves JG, McKay RD et al: Factors and their influence on regional cerebral blood flow during nonpulsatile cardiopulmonary bypass. Ann Thorac Surg 38:592–600, 1984

48. Miyamato K, Kawahima Y, Matsuda H et al: Optimal perfusion flow rate for the brain during deep hypothermic cardiopulmonary bypass at 20°C. J Thorac Cardiovasc Surg 92:1065–1070, 1986

49. Norwood WI, Norwood CR, Castaneda AR: Cerebral anoxia: Effect of deep hypothermia and pH. Surgery 86:203–210, 1979

50. Fox LS, Blackstone EH, Kirklin JW et al: Relationship of brain blood flow and oxygen consumption to perfusion flow rate during profound hypothermic cardiopulmonary bypass an experimental study. J Thorac Cardiovasc Surg 87:658–664, 1984

51. Somero GN, White FN: Enzymatic consequences under alpha stat regulation. In Rahn H, Prakash O (eds): Acid–Base Regulation and Body Temperature, pp. 55–80. Nijhoff, Boston, 1985

52. Aoki M, Nomura F, Stromski ME et al: Effects of pH strategy on recovery of piglet brain energetics after hypothermic circulatory arrest. Ann Thorac Surg 55:1093–2103.

53. Swain JA, McDonald TJ, Robbins RC et al: Relationship of cerebral and myocardial intracellular pH to blood pH during hypothermia. Am J Physiol 260:H1640–H1644.

54. Clark RE, Dietz DR, Miller JG: Continuous detection of microemboli during cardiopulmonary bypass in animals and man. Circulation 54:74–78, 1976

55. Orenstein JM, Sato N, Aaron B et al: Microemboli observed in deaths following cardiac surgery. Hum Pathol 13:1082–1090, 1982

56. Blauth CI, Arnold JV, Schulenberg WE et al: Cerebral microembolism during cardiopulmonary bypass. J Thorac Cardiovasc Surg 95:668–676, 1988

57. Deverall PB, Padayachee TS, Parson E et al: Ultrasound detection of microemboli in the middle cerebral artery during cardiopulmonary bypass surgery. Eur J Cardiothorac Surg 2:256–260, 1988

58. Greeley WJ, Kern FH, Ungerleider RM et al: Intramyocardial air causes right ventricular dysfunction after repair of a congenital heart defect. Anesthesiology 73:1042–1046, 1990

59. Moody DM, Bell MA, Challa VR et al: Brain microemboli during cardiac surgery or aortography. Ann Neurol 28:477–486, 1990

60. Blauth C, Smith P, Newman S et al: Retinal microembolism and neuro-psychiatric deficit following clinical cardiopulmonary bypass: Comparison of a membrane and a bubble oxygenator. Eur J Cardiothorac Surg 3: 135–139, 1989

61. Semb BKH, Pedersen T, Hatteland K et al: Doppler ultrasound estimation of bubble removal by various arterial line filters during extracorporeal circulation. Scand J Thorac Cardiovasc Surg 16:55–62, 1982

62. Young JA, Kisker CT, Doty DB: Adequate anticoagulation during cardiopulmonary bypass determined by activated clotting time and the appearance of fibrin monomer. Ann Thorac Surg 26:231–240, 1978

63. Newburger JW, Jonas RA, Wernovsky G et al: A comparison of the perioperative neurologic effects of hypothermic circulatory arrest versus low-flow cardiopulmonary bypass in infant heart surgery. N Engl J Med 329: 1057–1064, 1993

64. Bell C, Rimar S, Barash P: ST-segment changes consistent with myocardial ischemia in the neonate: A report of three cases. Anesthesiology 71: 601–604, 1989

65. Stegman T, Daniel W, Bellman L et al: Experimental coronary air embolism: Assessment of time course of myocardial ischemia and the protective effect of cardiopulmonary bypass. J Thorac Cardiovasc Surg 28: 141–145, 1980

66. Armon C, Deschamps C, Fealey RD et al: Hyperbaric treatment of cerebral air embolism sustained during an open-heart surgical procedure. Mayo Clin Proc 66:565–571, 1991

67. Chizzonite R, Zak R: Calcium-induced cell death: Susceptability of cardiac myocytes is age-dependent. Science 213:508–511, 1981

68. Julia PL, Kofsky ER, Buckberg GD et al: Studies of myocardial protection in the immature heart. I. Enhanced tolerance of immature vs adult myocardium to global ischemia with reference to metabolic differences. J Thorac Cardiovasc Surg 100:879–888, 1990

69. Hoerter J: Changes in the sensitivity to hypoxia and glucose deprivation in the isolated perfused rabbit heart during perinatal development. Pflugers Arch 303:1–6, 1976

70. Julia PL, Young HH, Buckberg GD et al: Studies of myocardial protection in the immature heart. II. Evidence for importance of amino acid metabolism in tolerance to ischemia. J Thorac Cardiovasc Surg 100:888–895, 1990

71. Mavroudis C, Ebert PA: Hemodilution causes decreased compliance in puppies. Circulation 58(suppl I):I154–I159, 1978

72. Jarmakani JM, Nagatomo T, Nakazawa M et al: Effect of hypoxia on myocardial high-energy phosphates in the neonatal mammalian heart. Am J Physiol 235:H475–H481, 1978

73. Julia PL, Kofsky ER, Buckberg GD et al: Studies of myocardial protection in the immature heart. III. Models of ischemic and hypoxic/ischemic injury in the immature puppy heart. J Thorac Cardiovasc Surg 101:14–19, 1991

74. Schwinn DA, Leone BJ, Spahn DR et al: Desensitization of myocardial beta-adrenergic receptors during cardiopulmonary bypass. Circulation 84:2559–2567, 1991

75. Schrantz D, Droege A, Broede A et al: Uncoupling of human cardiac beta-adrenoceptors during cardiopulmonary bypass with cardioplegic cardiac arrest. Circulation 87:422–426, 1993

76. Deal CW, Warden JC, Monk I: Effect of hypothermia on lung compliance. Thorax 25:105–109, 1970
77. Ashmore PG, Wakeford J, Harterre D: Pulmonary complications of profound hypothermia with circulatory arrest in the experimental animal. Can J Surg 7:93–96, 1964
78. Vincent RN, Lang P, Elixson M et al: Measurement of extravascular lung water in infants and children after cardiac surgery. Am J Cardiol 54: 161–165, 1984
79. McGowan FX Jr, Ikegami M, del Nido PJ et al: Cardiopulmonary bypass significantly reduces surfactant activity in children. J Thorac Cardiovasc Surg 106:968–977, 1993
80. Royall JA, Levin DL: Adult respiratory distress syndrome in pediatric patients. Clinical aspects, pathophysiology and mechanisms of lung injury. J Pediatr 112:169–180, 1988
81. Stanley TH, Philbin DM, Coggins CH: Fentanyl-oxygen anesthesia for coronary artery surgery: Cardiovascular and antidiuretic hormone responses. Can Anaesth Soc J 26:168–172, 1979
82. Stanley TH, Berman L, Gren O et al: Plasma catecholamine and cortisol responses to fentanyl-oxygen anesthesia for coronary artery operations. Anesthesiology 55:250–253, 1980
83. Taylor KM, Morton IL, Brown JJ et al: Hypertension and the renin angiotensin system following open heart surgery. J Thorac Cardiovasc Surg 74:840–845, 1977
84. Goodman TA, Gerard DF, Bernstein EF et al: The effects of pulseless perfusion on the distribution of renal cortical blood flow and renin. Surgery 80:31–39, 1976
85. German JC, Chalmers GS, Mukherjee D et al: Comparison of nonpulsatile and pulsatile extracorporeal circulation on renal tissue perfusion. Chest 61:65–68, 1972
86. Hilberman M, Myers BD, Carrie et al: Acute renal failure following cardiac surgery. J Thorac Cardiovasc Surg 77:880–888, 1979
87. Kron IL, Joob AW, Van Meter C: Acute renal failure in the cardiovascular surgical patient. Ann Thorac Surg 39:590–598, 1985
88. Hilberman M, Derby GC, Spencer RJ et al: Sequential pathophysiological changes characterizing the progression from renal dysfunction to acute renal failure following cardiac operation. J Thorac Cardiovasc Surg 79: 838–844, 1980
89. Gomez-Campdera FJ, Maroto-Alvaro E, Galinanes M et al: Acute renal failure associated with cardiac surgery. Child Nephrol Urol 9:138–143, 1988
90. Astrup J: Energy-requiring cell functions in the ischemic brain. J Neurosurg 56:482, 1982
91. Ericinska M, Silver IA: ATP and brain function. J Cereb Blood Flow Metab 9:2, 1989
92. Hansen AJ: Effect of anoxia on ion distribution in the brain. Physiol Rev 65:101, 1985
93. Norstrom CH, Siesko BK: Influence of phenobarbital on changes in the metabolites of the energy reserve of the cerebral cortex following complete ischemia. Acta Physiol Scand 104:271, 1978
94. Benveniste H, Drejer J, Schousboe A et al: Elevations of the extracellular concentrations of glutamate and aspartate in rat hippocampus during transient cerebral ischemia monitored by intracerebral microdialysis. J Neurochem 43:1369–1374, 1984

95. Hagberg J, Andersson P, Lacarewicz J et al: Extracellular adenosine, inosine, hypoxanthine, and xanthine in relation to tissue nucleotides and purines in rat striatum during transient ischemia. J Neurochem 49:227, 1987

96. Hagberg J, Andersson P, Kjellmer I et al: Extracellular overflow of glutamate, aspartate, GABA, and taurine in the cortex and basal ganglia of fetal lambs during hypoxia-ischemia. Neurosci Lett 78:311–317, 1987

97. Mutch WAC, Hansen AJ: Extracellular pH changes during spreading depression and cerebral ischemia: Mechanisms of brain pH regulation. J Cereb Blood Flow Metab 4:17, 1984

98. Hansen AJ, Zeuthen T: Extracellular ion concentrations during spreading depression and ischemia in the rat brain cortex. Acta Physiol Scand 113:437, 1981

99. Mies G, Paschen W: Regional changes of blood flow, glucose, and ATP content determined on brain sections during a single passage of spreading depression in rat brain cortex. Exp Neurol 84:249, 1984

100. Wieloch T, Harris R, Symon L et al: Influence of severe hypoglycemia on brain extracellular calcium and potassium activities, energy, and phospholipid metabolism. J Neurochem 43:160, 1984

101. Tang W, Sun GY: Effects of ischemia on free fatty acids and diacylglycerols in developing rat brain. J Dev Neurosci 3:51–56, 1985

102. Gaudet RJ, Alam I, Levine L: Accumulation of cyclooxygenase products of arachidonic acid metabolism in gerbil brain during reperfusion after bilateral common carotid artery occlusion. J Neurochem 35:653–658, 1980

103. Adesuyi SA, Cockrell CS, Gamache DA et al: Lipoxygenase metabolism of arachidonic acid in brain. J Neurochem 45:770, 1985

104. Moskowitz MA, Kiwak KJ, Hekimian K et al: Synthesis of compounds with properties of leukotrienes C4 and D4 in gerbil brains after ischemia and reperfusion. Science 224:886, 1984

105. Tullis RH, Rubin H: Calcium protects DNAseI from proteinase K: A new method for the removal of spin-trapped radicals in aqueous solutions of pyrimidine nucleosides and nucleotides. Reaction of the hydroxyl radical. Int J Radiat Biol 41:241, 1982

106. Ward JF, Blakeky WF, Joner EI: Mammalian cells are not killed by DNA single-strand breaks caused by hydroxyl radicals from hydrogen peroxide. Radiat Res 103:383, 1985.

107. Radford IR: The level of induced DNA double strand breakage correlates with cell killing after x-radiation. Int J Radiat Biol 48:45, 1985

108. Bryant PE: Enzymatic restriction of mammalian cell DNA: Evidence for double-strand breaks as potentially lethal lesions. Int J Rad Res 48:55, 1985

109. Guitierrez G: Cellular energy metabolism during hypoxia. Crit Care Med 19:619–626, 1991

110. Freeman BA, Crapo JD: Free radicals and tissue injury. Lab Invest 47:412, 1982

111. Norwood WI, Norwood CR, Ingwall JS et al: Hypothermic circulatory arrest: 31-phosphorus nuclear magnetic resonance of isolated perfused neonatal rat brain. J Thorac Cardiovasc Surg 78:823–830, 1979

112. Sutton LN, Clark BJ, Norwood CR: Global cerebral ischemia in piglets under conditions of mild and deep hypothermia. Stroke 22:1567–1573, 1991

113. Chopp M, Knight R, Tidwell CD et al: The metabolic effects of moderate hypothermia on global cerebral ischemia and recirculation in the cat:

Comparison to monothermia and hypothermia. J Cereb Blood Flow Metab 9:141, 1989

114. Stocker F, Hershkowitz N, Bossi E et al: Cerebral metabolic studies in situ by 31P-nuclear magnetic resonance after hypothermic circulatory arrest. Pediatr Res 20(9):867–871, 1986

115. Jonas RA: Experimental studies of hypothermic circulatory arrest and low flow bypass. Cardiol Young 3:299–307, 1993

116. Moskowitz MA, Meyer E, Wurtman RJ et al: Attenuation of catecholamine antagonists of the hypothermia that follows cerebral infarction in the gerbil. Life Sci 293:332, 1975

117. Rothman SM, Olney JW: Glutamate and the pathophysiology of hypoxic-ischemic brain damage. Ann Neurol 19:105, 1986

118. Globus MY, Ginsberg MD, Harik ST et al: Role of dopamine in ischemic striatal injury: Metabolic evidence. Neurology 37:1712, 1987

119. Globus MY, Ginsberg MD, Dietrich WD et al: Substantia nigra lesions protect against ischemic damage on the striatum. Neurosci Lett 80:251, 1987

120. Berntman L, Welsh FA, Harp JR: Cerebral protective effect of low grade hypothermia. Anesthesiology 55:495, 1981

121. Busto R, Dietrich WD, Globus MY et al: Small differences in the intra-ischemic brain temperature critically determine the extent of ischemic neuronal injury. J Cereb Blood Flow Metab 7:729, 1987

122. Rich TL, Langer GA: Calcium depletion in rabbit myocardium: Calcium paradox protection by hypothermia and cation substitution. Circ Res 51:131–141, 1982

123. Greeley WJ, Ungerleider RM, Kern FH et al: Effects of cardiopulmonary bypass on cerebral blood flow in neonates, infants and children. Circulation 80(suppl I):I-209–I-215, 1989

124. Murkin JM, Farrar JK, Tweed WA et al: Cerebral autoregulation and flow/metabolic coupling during cardiopulmonary bypass. Anesth Analg 66:825–832, 1987

125. Greeley WJ, Ungerleider RM, Smith LR et al: The effect of deep hypothermic cardiopulmonary bypass and total circulatory arrest on cerebral blood flow in infants and children. J Thorac Cardiovasc Surg 97:737–745, 1989

126. Kern FH, Ungerleider RM, Quill TJ et al: Cerebral blood flow response to changes in $PaCO_2$ during hypothermic cardiopulmonary bypass in children. J Thorac Cardiovasc Surg 101:618–622, 1991

127. Kern FH, Ungerleider RM, Reves JG et al: The effects of altering pump flow rate on cerebral blood flow and metabolism in neonates, infants and children. Ann Thorac Surg, in press, 1995

128. Michenfelder JD: The awake brain. In Michenfelder JD (ed): Anesthesia and the Brain, pp. 7–8. New York, Churchill Livingstone, 1988

129. Michenfelder JD, Theye RA: Hypothermia: Effect of canine brain and whole-body metabolism. Anesthesiology 29:1107, 1968

130. Bering EA Jr: Effect of body temperature change on cerebral oxygen consumption during hypothermia. Am J Physiol 200:417, 1961

131. Croughwell N, Smith LR, Quill T et al: The effect of temperature on cerebral metabolism and blood flow in adults during cardiopulmonary bypass. J Thorac Cardiovasc Surg 103:549, 1993

132. Kern FH, Jonas RA, Mayer JE et al: Temperature monitoring during infant CPB: Does it predict efficient brain cooling? Ann Thorac Surg 54:749–754, 1992

133. Scheinberg P, Stead EA: The cerebral blood flow in male subjects as measured by the nitrous technique: Normal values for blood flow, oxygen utilization, glucose utilization, and peripheral resistance with observations on the effect of lilting and anxiety. J Clin Invest 28:1163–1168, 1949
134. Rosenberg AA, Jones MD, Traystman RJ et al: Response of cerebral blood flow to changes in PCO_2 in fetal, newborn and adult sheep. Am J Physiol 242(5):H862–H866, 1982
135. Mault JR, Ohtake S, Klingensmith ME et al: Cerebral metabolism and circulatory arrest: Effects of duration and strategies for protection. Ann Thorac Surg 55:57–64, 1993
136. Mault JR, Whitaker EG, Heinle JS et al: Intermittent perfusion during hypothermic circulatory arrest: A new and effective technique for cerebral protection. In Surgical Forum. American College of Surgeons, Clinical Congress, 1992
137. Prough DS, Stump DA, Roy RC et al: Response of cerebral blood flow to changes in carbon dioxide tension during hypothermic cardiopulmonary bypass. Anesthesiology 64:576–581, 1986
138. Slogoff S, Girgis KZ, Keats AS: Etiologic factors in neuropsychiatric complications associated with cardiopulmonary bypass. Anesth Analg 61:903–911, 1982
139. Glauser TA, Rorke LB, Weinberg PM et al: Acquired neuropathologic lesions associated with the hypoplastic left heart syndrome. Pediatrics 85(6):991–1000, 1990
140. Bashein G, Townes BD, Nessly BS et al: A randomized study of carbon dioxide management during hypothermic cardiopulmonary bypass. Anesthesiology 72:7–15, 1990
141. Hindman BJ: Cerebral physiology of hypothermia during bypass. Cardiol Young 3:273–278, 1993
142. Swan H: The importance of acid–base management for cardiac and cerebral preservation during open heart operations. Surg Gynecol Obstet 158:391–414, 1984
143. Siesjo BK, Bendek G, Koide T et al: Influence of acidosis on lipid peroxidation in brain tissue in vitro. J Cereb Blood Flow Metab 5:253, 1985
144. Bellinger PC, Wernovsky G, Rappaport LA et al: Rapid cooling of infants on cardiopulmonary bypass adversely affects later cognitive function. Circulation 78(suppl II):II-358–II-363
145. Kern FH, Ungerleider RM, Schulman SR et al: Comparison of two strategies of CPB cooling on jugular venous oxygen saturation. Ann Thorac Surg, in press, 1995
146. Busto R, Mordecai Y-T, Dietrich D et al: Effects of mild hypothermia on brain ischemia. Stroke 20(7):904–910, 1989
147. Okada Y, Tanimoto M, Yoneda K: The protective effect of hypothermia on reversibility in the neuronal function of the hippocampal slice during long lasting anoxia. Neurosci Lett 84:277–282, 1988
148. Hansen NB, Brubakk AM, Bratlid D et al: The effects of variations in $PaCO_2$ in brain blood flow and cardiac output in the newborn piglet. Pediatr Res 18(11):1132–1136, 1984
149. Skaryak LA, Chai PJ, Kern FH et al: Combining alpha and pH stat blood gas strategy prior to circulatory arrest provides optimal recovery of cerebral metabolism. Circulation, suppl I, 1993
150. Spach MS, Serwer GA, Anderson PAW et al: Pulsatile aortopulmonary pressure-flow dynamics of patent ductus arteriosus in patients with various hemodynamic states. Circulation 61:110–122, 1980

151. Brunberg JA, Doty DB, Reilly EL: Choreoathetosis in infants following cardiac surgery with deep hypothermia and circulatory arrest. J Pediatr 84(2):232–235, 1974
152. Egerton N, Egerton WS, Kay JH: Neurologic changes following profound hypothermia. Ann Surg 157:366–382, 1963
153. Bachet J, Guilmet D, Goudot B et al: "Cold Cerebroplegia": A new technique of cerebral protection during surgery of the transverse aortic arch. In 70th Annual Meeting of the American Association for Thoracic Surgery. Toronto, 1990
154. Salama A, Mueller-Eckhardt C: Delayed hemolytic transfusion reactions. Evidence for complement activation involving allogenic autologous red cells. Transfusion 214:188–193, 1984
155. Ratcliffe JM, Elliott MJ, Wyse RKH et al: The metabolic load of stored blood. Implications for major transfusion in infants. Arch Dis Child 61: 1208–1214, 1986
156. Hepps SA, Roe BR, Wright RR et al: Amelioration of the postperfusion syndrome with haemodilution and low molecular weight dextran. Surgery 54:32–43, 1963
157. Utley JR, Wachtel C, Cain RB et al: Effects of hypothermia, hemodilution and pump oxygenation on organ water content, blood flow, oxygen delivery and renal function. Ann Thorac Surg 31:121–133, 1981
158. Kawashima Y, Yamamoto Z, Manabe H: Safe limits of hemodilution in cardiopulmonary bypass. Surgery 76:391–397, 1974
159. Henling CE, Carmichael MJ, Keats AS et al: Cardiac operation for congenital heart disease in children of Jehovah's Witnesses. J Thorac Cardiovasc Surg 89:914–920, 1985
160. Leone BJ, Spahn DR, McRae RL et al: Effects of hemodilution and anesthesia on regional function of compromised myocardium. Anesthesiology 73:A596, 1990
161. VanOerversen W, Kazatchkine MD, Descamp-Latscha et al: Deleterious effects of cardiopulmonary bypass: A prospective study of bubble versus membrane oxygenators. J Thorac Cardiovasc Surg 89:888–899, 1985
162. Horton AM, Butt W: Pump-induced haemolysis: Is the constrained vortex pump better or worse than the roller pump? Perfusion 7:103–108, 1992
163. Becker AE, Caruso G: Congenital heart disease—a morphologist's view on myocardial dysfunction. In LG, Becker AE, Marcelleti C, Anderson RH (eds): Paediatric Cardiology. Edinburgh, Churchill Livingstone, 1981
164. Oshita S, Uchimoto R, Oka H et al: Correlation between arterial blood pressure and oxygenation in tetralogy of Fallot. J Cardiovasc Anesth 3(5): 597–600, 1989
165. Severinghaus JW, Spellman BA: Pulse oximeter failure thresholds in hypotension and vasoconstriction. Anesthesiology 73:532–537, 1990
166. Gold JP, Jonas RA, Lang P et al: Transthoracic intracardiac monitoring lines in pediatric surgical patients: A ten year experience. Ann Thorac Surg 42:185, 1986
167. Ungerleider RM, Greeley WJ, Sheikh KH et al: The use of intraoperative echo with Doppler color flow imaging to predict outcome after repair of congenital cardiac defects. Ann Surg 210(4):526, 1989
168. Ungerleider RM, Greeley WJ, Sheikh KH et al: Routine use of intraoperative epicardial echo and Doppler color flow imaging to guide and evaluate repair of congenital heart lesions: A prospective study. J Thorac Cardiovasc Surg 100(2):297, 1990

169. Muhiudeen IA, Roberson DA, Silverman NH et al: Intraoperative echocardiography in infants and children with congenital cardiac shunt lesions—transesophageal versus epicardial echocardiography. J Am Coll Cardiol 16:7–12, 1990
170. Muhiudeen IA, Roberson DA, Silverman NH et al: Intraoperative echocardiography for evaluation of congenital heart defects in infants and children. Anesthesiology 76:165–172, 1992
171. Bohn DJ, Piorier CS, Edmonds JF et al: Hemodynamic effects of dobutamine after cardiopulmonary bypass in children. Crit Care Med 8: 367–342, 1980
172. Bohn DJ, Poirer CS, Edmonds JF et al: Efficacy of dopamine, dobutamine, and epinephrine during emergence from cardiopulmonary bypass in children. Crit Care Med 8:367–372, 1980
173. Lawless S, Burckart G, Diven W et al: Amrinone pharmacokinetics in neonates and infants. J Clin Pharmacol 28:283, 1988
174. Hines R, Barash PG: Right ventricular failure. In Kaplan JA (ed): Cardiac Anesthesia, 2nd ed., vol. 2. New York, Grune & Stratton, 1987
175. Drummond WH, Gregory GA, Heyman MA et al: The independent effects of hyperventilation, tolazoline, and dopamine in infants with persistant pulmonary hypertension. J Pediatr 98:603–608, 1981
176. Morray JP, Lynn AM, Mansfield PB: Effects of pH and PCO_2 on pulmonary and systemic hemodynamics after surgery in children with congenital heart disease and pulmonary hypertension. J Pediatr 113:474, 1988
177. Lyrene RK, Welch KA, Godoy G et al: Alkalosis attenuates hypoxic pulmonary vasoconstriction in neonatal lambs. Pediatr Res 19(12):1268, 1985
178. Rudolph AM, Yuan S: Response of the pulmonary vasculature to hypoxia and $H+$ ion concentration changes. J Clin Invest 45:399, 1966
179. Zapletal A, Paul T, Samenek M: Pulmonary elasticity in children and adolescents. J Appl Physiol 40:953, 1976
180. Mansell A, Bryan AC: Airway closure in children. J Appl Physiol 33:711, 1972
181. Hammon JW, Wolfe WG, Moran JF et al: The effect of positive end expiratory pressure on regional ventilation and perfusion in the normal and injured primate lung. J Thorac Cardiovasc Surg 72:680, 1976
182. Jenkins J, Lynn A, Edmonds J et al: Effects of mechanical ventilation on cardiopulmonary function in children after open-heart surgery. Crit Care Med 13:77–80, 1985
183. Meliones JN, Bove EL, Dekeon MK et al: High-frequency jet ventilation improves cardiac function after the Fontan procedure. Circulation 84(suppl III):III-364–III-368, 1991
184. Roberts JD, Lang P, Bigatello LM et al: Inhaled nitric oxide in congenital heart disease. Circulation 87:447–453, 1993
185. Girard C, Lehot JJ, Clerc J et al: Inhaled nitric oxide (NO) in pulmonary hypertension following mitral valve replacement. Anesthesiology 75: A984, 1991
186. Roberts JD, Chen TY, Kawai N et al: Inhaled nitric oxide reverses pulmonary vasoconstriction in the hypoxic and acidotic newborn lamb. Circ Res 72:246–254, 1993
187. Benotti JR, Grossman W, Braunwald E et al: Effects of amrinone on myocardial energy metabolism and hemodynamics in patients with severe congestive heart failure due to coronary disease. Circulation 62:28–34, 1980

188. Hess W, Arnold B, Veit S: The hemodynamic effects of amrinone in patients with mitral stenosis and pulmonary hypertension. Eur Heart J 7: 800–807, 1986

189. Konstam MA, Cohen SR, Salem DN et al: Effect of amrinone on right ventricular function: Predominance of afterload reduction. Circulation 74: 359–366, 1986

190. Wessel DL, Triedman JK, Wernovsky G et al: Pulmonary and systemic hemodynamics of amrinone in neonates following cardiopulmonary bypass. Circulation suppl II(80):II488, 1989

191. Schwartz DA, Grove FL, Horowitz LD: Effect of isoproterenol on regional myocardial perfusion and tissue oxygenation in acute myocardial infarction. Am Heart J 97:339, 1979

192. Molloy DW: Effects of noradrenaline and isoproterenol on cardiopulmonary function in a canine model of acute pulmonary hypertension. Chest 88:432, 1985

193. D'ambra M, LaRaia P, Phellan D et al: A new therapy for refractory right heart failure and pulmonary hypertension after mitral valve replacement. J Thorac Cardiovasc Surg 89:567–572, 1985

194. Greeley WJ, Kern FH: Anesthesia for pediatric cardiac surgery. In Miller RD (ed): Anesthesia, pp. 1693–1736. New York, Churchill Livingstone, 1990

195. Vlahakes GJ, Turley K, Hoffman JIE: The pathophysiology of failure in right ventricular hypertension: Hemodynamic and biological correlations. Circulation 63:87–92, 1980

196. Ungerleider RM, Greeley WJ, Kanter RJ et al: The learning curve for intraoperative echocardiography during congenital heart surgery. Ann Thorac Surg 54:691–698, 1992

197. Naik SK, Knight A, Elliott MJ: A prospective randomized study of a modified technique of ultrafiltration during pediatric open-heart surgery. Circulation 84(suppl III):III-422–III-431, 1991

198. Naik SK, Knight A, Elliot MJ: A successful modification of ultrafiltration for cardiopulmonary bypass in children. Perfusion 6:41–50, 1991

Philippe Pouard
Didier Journois
William J. Greeley

Hemofiltration and Pediatric Cardiac

4 Surgery

Pediatric cardiopulmonary bypass (CPB) often results in increased capillary permeability and increased total body water (TBW). The increase in TBW may lead to tissue edema and multiple organ dysfunction, including of the brain, heart, and lungs. The small blood volume of children, compared to the priming volume of the CPB circuit, results in significant hemodilution. Exposure of the patient's blood to the foreign surface of the oxygenator results in a significant inflammatory response that may exacerbate the increase in TBW. CPB is known to induce a capillary leak syndrome that can lead to fluid overload and organ dysfunction. This process is associated with a systemic inflammatory response that may lead to severe postoperative complications.[1,2] This hormonal and metabolic stress response to CPB is particularly exacerbated in the neonate during pediatric CPB for congenital heart surgery, due to organ maturational features, the specific type of surgical repair, and the special extracorporeal techniques used, such as deep hypothermic circulatory arrest.

A variety of techniques have been developed to reverse tissue edema and hemodilution after CPB, including ultrafiltration during CPB, postoperative peritoneal dialysis, postoperative continuous arteriovenous hemofiltration, aggressive use of diuretics postoperatively, and infusion of salvaged circuit volume. In the pediatric population, ultrafiltration and cell centrifugation during CPB are restricted by the

Perioperative Management of the Patient with Congenital Heart Disease, edited by William J. Greeley. Williams & Wilkins, Baltimore © 1996.

volume in the venous reservoir and provide only a limited ability to remove excess water and reverse hemodilution.

Hemofiltration is a technique that uses the convection process to remove water and some low molecular weight substances from plasma under a hydrostatic pressure gradient. Because the hemodilution effects of CPB are especially pronounced in children due to a disproportionately large priming volume of the CPB circuit, the potential benefit of hemofiltration could be very significant in these small patients. This technique has effectively been used after CPB termination in children and appears to be an effective therapy to reduce the amount of accumulated tissue water and to concentrate the blood at the end of CPB.[3] More recently, the use of hemofiltration after CPB has been associated with a marked improvement in hemodynamics,[4,5] cardiac contractility[2] and oxygenation,[2,6,7] and a reduction in postoperative blood loss and duration of mechanical ventilation.[3,4] These beneficial effects of hemofiltration were initially attributed to a reduction in tissue edema.[3] However, recent experimental studies[6,7] and clinical investigations have demonstrated the removal of several major inflammatory mediators by hemofiltration,[2,4] suggesting that water removal is not the only mechanism that improves outcome.

PHYSIOLOGICAL FLUID HOMEOSTASIS IN THE NEONATE

At birth, neonates have an interstitial water excess that will spontaneously decrease approximately 10% within the first 3 days of life. During the neonatal period, interstitial water represents 55% of TBW, as compared to 35% TBW seen in adult patients. In addition to excess interstitial fluid, the neonate has immature renal function in the first 2 months of life. At birth, glomerular filtration is approximately 10 ml/m^2/minute, increases rapidly to 20 ml/m^2/minute during the second week of life, and reaches 45 to 120 ml/m^2/minute at the end of the second month.[8] Renal tubular function is also impaired, and that results in a reduced concentrating capacity, compared to that in adult patients. Urinary osmolarity can only be increased from 40 mOsm/liter to 800 mOsm/liter (1400 mOsm/liter in adults and only 600 mOsm/liter in premature baby). Renal dilutional capacity follows a similar trend but at less a rate of reduction. Bicarbonate reabsorption is also impaired. Thus, the immature kidney in young patients is unable to excrete a fluid or acid overload rapidly.

The physiological interstitial water excess in normal neonates is increased as a result of CPB. CPB induces fluid retention because of activation of the systemic inflammatory response due to the exposure of blood elements to nonendothelialized surfaces. This situation is further exacerbated by the use of hemodilution, deep hypothermia, non-pulsatile pump flow, low pump flow, and impaired intraoperative renal function. The use of prostaglandin E_1 in the preoperative period also increases fluid retention. Intraoperatively, interstitial tissue edema may be increased by some deleterious events, such as excessive water intake (cardioplegic solutions), acute dilatation of left atrium, or a displacement of the venous cannulae that will create caval obstruction and decrease venous drainage.

To summarize, the physiological fluid excess of the neonate, renal immaturity, and biological and mechanical side effects of CPB all lead to a potentially deleterious interstitial fluid accumulation. This interstitial edema may result in organ dysfunction (e.g., impede pulmonary gas exchange, delay separation from mechanical ventilation, impair hemostasis, decrease myocardial contractility, and decrease cerebral metabolic recovery) and increase morbidity and mortality.

Under most circumstances, diuretic administration at the end of CPB and in the ICU remains the only therapy. Diuretic therapy is often limiting and may induce severe metabolic disorders and uncontrollable diuresis. Moreover, this approach is only helpful when hemodynamic status is appropriate, and diuretics do not prevent interstitial edema. In the postoperative period, when myocardial function is impaired for any reason, low cardiac output will lead to increased interstitial edema due to decreased renal perfusion and secondary aldosterone secretion, decreased oxygen delivery to tissues, and aggravation of low cardiac output. Therefore, after CPB, hemofiltration appears to have value as a protective and preventative therapy.

THE HEMOFILTRATION CIRCUIT

Conventional Hemofiltration

With *conventional* hemofiltration, filtration occurs during the rewarming phase of CPB, before actual separation. The hemofiltration unit can be set up at different places on the CPB circuit. The simplest setup removes blood at the vent of the arterial filter, directs blood through the hemofilter, and reinfuses it in the cardiotomy reservoir (Fig. 4–1). The advantage of this setup is the use of the arterial pump as the driving force of the filtration pressure. The main disadvantage is the relation between the perfusion pressure and the hemofiltration flow. When the hemofiltration flow increases, at a constant pump flow, blood flow in the patient decreases and, consequently, perfusion pressure decreases. Immediately before terminating hemofiltration, it is necessary to decrease the pump flow to avoid an acute dilatation of

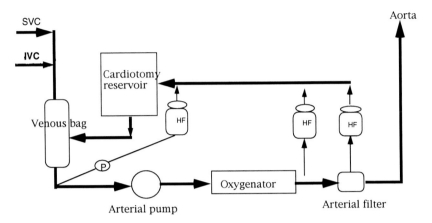

FIGURE 4–1. Hemofilter (HF) set up in closed circuits for conventional hemofiltration. *SVC*, superior vena cava; *IVC*, inferior vena cava; *HF*, hemofilter; *P*, pump.

the heart because of a sudden increase of blood flow in the arterial line.

The inlet line of the hemofilter can also be connected at a cardioplegia outlet of the gas exchange. The placement of the inlet line of the hemofilter on the venous return line is possible but another pump will be needed as a driving force (Fig. 4–1).

Modified Hemofiltration

With *modified* hemofiltration, filtration occurs after separation from CPB. Modified hemofiltration is usually continued for 10 to 15 minutes immediately after bypass. The hemofilter is placed on a shunt, excluding the gas exchanger on the main CPB circuit. The blood is then slowly directed through the hemofilter from the arterial canula to a small vent inserted into the right atrium.[9] This circuit needs a roller pump at the inlet of the ultrafilter. Hemofiltration is carried out smoothly at a flow rate between 100 and 200 ml/minute after cessation of CPB. The arterial pump can be used during hemofiltration to deliver volume from the venous reservoir if the patient becomes hypotensive. This fluid passes through the oxygenator to the inlet of the hemofilter and does not enter the aortic line when the flow is less than 150 ml/minute[10] (Fig. 4–2). Monitoring a left atrial pressure line, if available, is often a very useful method of monitoring filling pressure during modified ultrafiltration.

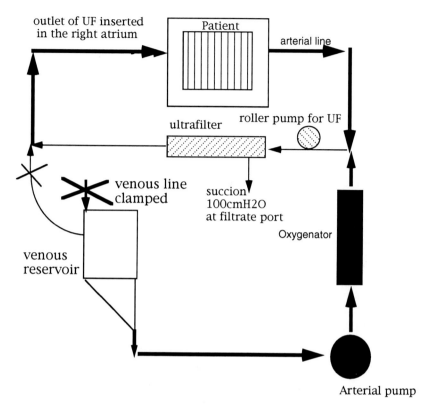

FIGURE 4–2. Circuit used for modified ultrafiltration. *(Reproduced with permission from Elliott MJ. Ann Thorac Surg 56:1518–1522, 1993)*

Careful attention to the patient's volume status is essential to maintain hemodynamic stability during modified hemofiltration. The central venous pressure (CVP) or left atrial pressure (LAP) can be maintained at appropriate levels by adjusting the flow rates of the arterial and modified hemofiltration pumps. Generally, the modified hemofiltration pump is maintained at a set flow rate of 15 to 20 ml/kg/minute. When the CVP or LAP drops, the arterial pump flow rate is slightly increased from the baseline flow rate. If the CVP or LAP is higher than desired, then the arterial pump flow rate is decreased or stopped. The arterial pump flow rate should not exceed the modified hemofiltration pump flow rate unless emergency rapid volume replacement is necessary, and before resuming antegrade flow through the aortic cannula, the arterial line should be carefully inspected for the presence of air. The patient's hematocrit is measured from arterial blood samples every 5 minutes during modified hemofiltration and after completion of modified hemofiltration.

HEMOFILTERS

There are many hemofilters available. The choice of an adequate filter is a key aspect of the technique. There is always a balance between the hemofiltration flow needed, which is dependent on the body surface area of the patient, and the priming volume of the hemofiltration circuit. The CPB circuits for neonates are usually primed with 350 to 450 ml of fluids, and it is reasonable not to increase this volume by more than 10%. Hemofiltration circuits primed with 20 to 30 ml seem to be adequate. For pediatric cardiac surgery, there is no particular advantage of the various fibers (polysulfone, polyamide, or polyacrylonitrile). Nevertheless, the use of polyacrilonitrile hemofilters may be preferred, because this filter is known to induce less complement activation than the polysulfone hemofilters and to adsorb complement fragments and precursors onto the membrane surface, thereby lowering complement levels.[11,12]

EFFECTS OF CONVENTIONAL AND MODIFIED HEMOFILTRATION

Effects on Ventilation

A reduction in the duration of mechanical ventilation and an increase in early postoperative PaO_2 has been reported after hemofiltration during correction of tetralogy of Fallot.[4] This improvement in oxygenation is likely to be mediated by water removal.[3] Nevertheless, net fluid balance seems to be a poor predictor of postoperative chest radiograph changes.[15] The beneficial effects of vasoactive substance removal by hemofiltration on pulmonary function has been demonstrated.[6] Journois et al.[4] have observed a correlation between C3a and C5a levels at the end of rewarming and in postoperative PaO_2, demonstrating the importance of modifying the inflammatory reaction and influencing the postoperative recovery of pulmonary function.[4]

Effects on Hemoconcentration and Hemostasis

Protein hemoconcentration has been reported in children when hemofiltration is performed either after CPB or in the postoperative period.[3,10,16,17] A 5 to 10% hemoconcentration effect of coagulation factors has been observed with conventional hemofiltration. Examining the hemoconcentration, the technique described by Naik et al.,[3] which ultrafilters exclusively the patient's blood volume and not the volume of the CPB circuit, is likely to be more efficient than conventional hemofiltration. Modified hemofiltration avoids the relatively ineffective filtration of the CPB circuit.[4] Therefore, modified ultrafiltration's benefit is maximal when a large difference exists between patient blood volume and CPB circuit priming volume (i.e., in younger children). Conventional hemofiltration only provides a limited increase in coagulation factor concentrations and no change in platelet count.[4] These results suggest that, when hemofiltration is performed during rewarming, its effects on postoperative bleeding are unlikely to be solely explained by hemoconcentration. Nevertheless, the use of hemofiltration during the rewarming period has the potential advantage of adjusting hematocrit and protein level.

Effects on Cardiovascular Performance

A significant increase in mean arterial pressure (MAP) has been observed after conventional hemofiltration,[4] establishing a positive correlation between MAP increase and the UF to TBV ratio (the ratio of ultrafiltrate volume to the estimated total blood volume). This finding supports the notion that withdrawal of ultrafiltrate is correlated with blood pressure improvement. The mechanism by which blood pressure improves remains uncertain. It is possible to speculate that hemofiltration may improve the elimination of some vasoactive substances that have a negative inotropic effect[18] or reduce myocardial water content, thereby improving cardiac output. This later hypothesis is supported by some recent findings that demonstrate a reduction in myocardial wall volume associated with an improvement of the left ventricle diastolic function produced by hemofiltration.[10] The benefit of blood pressure improvement is questionable, because hemoconcentration increases hematocrit and should increase blood viscosity, leading to increased systemic vascular resistance. Nonetheless, Naik et al. demonstrated that the overall effect of hemofiltration is an increase in cardiac index, blood pressure and systemic vascular resistance associated with a decrease in heart rate and pulmonary vascular resistance.[5]

Effects on Complement Fragments

Andreasson et al. have confirmed the activation of the complement cascade by CPB during pediatric cardiac surgery.[1] Moreover, these authors performed hemofiltration after CPB and noticed high concentrations of C3a and C5a in the ultrafiltrate. The lack of a control group in their study limited the interpretation of their data. Journois et al.[4] observed that levels of C3a and C5a in their own study were higher than those in adult patients in a previous report. This could be due to a heightened inflammatory response to CPB known to occur in children.[19] They observed that hemofiltration actually reduces the plasma concentrations of these complement components in such a way that the effects of C3a and C5a removal could delay cytokine release induced by these complement fragments, which was described by Haeffner-Cavaillon et al.[20] The C3a fragment triggers the formation of a terminal complement complex that stimulates neutrophil degranulation. The C3a fragment deposits on pulmonary vascular endothelium during CPB mediates increased expression of neutrophil CD18 adhesion protein and neutrophil sequestration.[21] A reduction of the postperfusion syndrome has been observed after administration of an inhibitor of complement activation, suggesting that this component is responsible for a large part of the syndrome.[22] Additional complement activation produced by the hemofiltration circuit may occur during the use of hemofiltration membranes.[12]

Effects on Cytokine Release

The numerous similarities between post-CPB morbidity and sepsis syndrome have led several groups to investigate cytokine release during and after CPB.[23,24] The elimination of TNFa and IL-1b by continuous hemofiltration[25] and the beneficial effects of continuous hemofiltration on cardiac and pulmonary function during sepsis states have been reported.[6,7,18] The volume of daily ultrafiltrate appears to influence organ function improvement during sepsis.[26,27]

Several reports have demonstrated that TNF, IL-6, and IL-8 release are stimulated by CPB in adults[20] and even more demonstrably in children.[2,13] The results of Millar et al.[2] and Journois et al.[4] show that hemofiltration, performed during the late phase of rewarming, is able to reduce the concentrations of IL-6 and TNFa. These substances that are removed from plasma by hemofiltration are not only removed by convection. Barrera et al. showed that incubation of polyacrilonitrile membrane fragments with radiolabeled IL-1b or TNF yielded a significant binding of both cytokines to the membrane. Removal was most marked in the first minutes, suggesting saturation of the membrane.[28] Therefore, cytokine binding on the hemofilter membrane may be a mechanism to explain the paradoxical lack of correlation between cytokine reduction and UF/TBV that we observed, as well as a correlation between cytokine level reduction and ultrafiltrate duration.

The IL-1b release is well documented in patients undergoing sequential hemodialysis[29,30] and occurs 20 hours later after exposure to CPB in adult cardiac surgery patients.[20] This delay could be explained by the fact that IL-1b release is triggered by complement activation.[31] Interleukin-8 is suspected of being a trigger of neutrophil-induced endothelial injury and, therefore, of being responsible for some of the postoperative CPB adverse effects.[13] The correlation between IL-8 release and the length of CPB has been demonstrated.[13] The results reported by Journois et al. confirm that IL-8 release is present during rewarming and that IL-8 is poorly eliminated by hemofiltration with a polysulfone membrane.[4] One reason may be that IL-8 is significantly bound by red cells; therefore, little is free to be filtered.[32]

DOES HEMOFILTRATION INDUCE SIDE EFFECTS?

Hopeck et al. reported no additional hemolysis when using hemofiltration during CPB.[33] Hemofiltration had no adverse effect on anesthetic or surgical techniques. The anesthetic agents are subject to high-protein binding,[34] and drug levels remained in the high therapeutic range,[35] even after large volume hemofiltration (D. Journois and P. Pouard, unpublished data).

The filtration of heparin has been very controversial and depends on the type of the hemofilter. The new membranes (polysulfone, polyamide, or polyacrylonitrile) filtrate a very small amount of heparin and only during the first minutes of use. Even if the size of the molecule does not prevent filtration, the electrical charge of heparin promotes its interaction with proteins that quickly coat the membrane and, therefore, act against its elimination. If the membrane is rinsed with a high volume of heparinized saline solution, heparin adsorption is rapidly saturated. After high-volume hemofiltration, a slight metabolic acidosis may appear. Sodium bicarbonate will be given carefully, so as not to induce hypernatremia. Aprotinin is highly removed by hemofiltration. Sixty to eighty percent of plasma aprotinin concentrations can be measured in the filtrate.[36]

Patient cooling during the MUF process has been observed, and the following steps can be taken to minimize this problem: (1) Patients should be fully warmed (37°C rectal) before termination of CPB. (2) the MUF circuit should be prewarmed by recirculating warm blood through the hemoconcentrator. (3) The MUF infusion cannula should be made as short as possible and (4) The operating-room temperature increased.

MODIFIED OR CONVENTIONAL TECHNIQUE: WHEN TO HEMOFILTRATE

Conventional hemofiltration is performed during rewarming of CPB. Although hemofiltration is able to eliminate several cytokines from blood, it may be more meaningful to perform this technique during rewarming to eliminate the early precursors of the inflammatory response, such as TNFa and complement fractions. There is currently some evidence that maximal complement and cytokine release coincide with the period of rewarming.[13,14] This preferential timing in cytokine release and hemofiltration use may justify the use of hemofiltration throughout the rewarming period, rather than only after CPB weaning. This technique may be a superior method of removing cytokines and complement fragments, compared to the modified hemofiltration technique, which is performed after CPB weaning. The modified hemofiltration technique seems to be more efficient with respect to water removal, fluid balance control, and hemoconcentration when used after CPB.

CONCLUSION

In conclusion, both techniques, conventional and modified hemofiltration, have been used successfully and enhance recovery from the deleterious effects of CPB. Recent studies have shown that hemofiltration limits positive water balance, decreases interstitial edema, improves organ function, and removes some major inflammatory mediators. Clinical use of this technique can be safely accomplished with appropriate circuit modifications and training and can result in improved patient outcome.

References

1. Andreasson S, Göthberg S, Berggren H, Bengtsson A, Eriksson E, Risberg B: Hemofiltration modifies complement activation after extracorporeal circulation in infants. Ann Thorac Surg 56:1515–1517, 1993
2. Millar AB, Armstrong L, van der Linden J, Moat N, Ekroth R, Westwick J, Scallan M, Lincoln C: Cytokine production and hemofiltration in children undergoing cardiopulmonary bypass. Ann Thorac Surg 56: 1499–1502, 1993
3. Naik SK, Knight A, Elliott M: A prospective randomized study of a modified technique of ultrafiltration during pediatric open-heart surgery. Circulation 84:422–431, 1991
4. Journois D, Pouard P, Greeley WJ, Mauriat P, Vouhé P, Safran D: Hemofiltration during cardiopulmonary bypass in pediatric cardiac surgery:

Effects on hemostasis, cytokines and complement components. Anesthesiology 81:1181–1189, 1994

5. Naik SK, Balaji S, Elliott MJ: Modified ultrafiltration improves hemodynamics after cardiopulmonary bypass in children. J Am Coll Cardiol 19: 37A, 1992

6. Stein B, Pfenninger E, Grunert A, Schmitz JE, Deller A, Kocher F: The consequences of continuous haemofiltration on lung mechanics and extravascular lung water in a porcine endotoxic shock model. Inten Care Med 17:293–298, 1991

7. Stein B, Pfenninger E, Grunert A, Schmitz JE, Hudde M: Influence of continuous haemofiltration on haemodynamics and central blood volume in experimental endotoxic shock. Intensive Care Med 16:494–499, 1990

8. Guignard JP: Renal function in the newborn infant. Pediatr Clin North Am 29:777–787, 1982

9. Naik SK, Knight A, Elliott MJ: A successful modification of ultrafiltration for cardiopulmonary bypass in children. Perfusion 6:41–50, 1991

10. Elliott MJ: Ultrafiltration and modified ultrafiltration in pediatric open heart operations. Ann Thorac Surg 56:1518–1522, 1993

11. Pascual M, Schifferli JA: Adsorption of complement factor D by polyacrylonitrile dialysis membranes. Kidney Int 43:903–911, 1993

12. Mulvihill J, Cazenave JP, Mazzucotelli JP, Crost T, Collier C, Renaux JL, Pusineri C: Minimodule dialyser for quantitative ex vivo evaluation of membrane haemocompatibility in humans: Comparison of acrylonitrile copolymer, cuprophan and polysulphone hollow fibres. Biomaterials 13: 527–536, 1992

13. Finn A, Naik S, Klein N, Levinsky RJ, Strobel S, Elliott M: Interleukin-8 release and neutrophil degranulation after pediatric cardiopulmonary bypass. J Thorac Cardiovasc Surg 105:234–241, 1993

14. Andreasson S, Göthberg S, Berggren H, Bengtsson A, Eriksson E, Risberg B: Hemofiltration modifies complement activation after extracorporeal circulation in infants. Ann Thorac Surg 56:1515–1517, 1993

15. Emhardt JD, Moorthy SS, Brown JW, Cohen MD, Wagner W Jr.: Chest radiograph changes after cardiopulmonary bypass in children. J Cardiovasc Surg 32:314–317, 1991

16. Zobel G, Stein JI, Kuttnig M, Beitzke A, Metzler H, Rigler B: Continuous extracorporeal fluid removal in children with low cardiac output after cardiac operations. J Thorac Cardiovasc Surg 101:593–597, 1991

17. Paret G, Cohen AJ, Bohn DJ, Edwards H, Taylor R, Geary D, Williams WG: Continuous arteriovenous hemofiltration after cardiac operations in infants and children. J Thorac Cardiovasc Surg 104:1225–1230, 1992

18. Gomez A, Wang R, Unruh H, Light RB, Bose D, Chau T, Correa E, Mink S: Hemofiltration reverses left ventricular dysfunction during sepsis in dogs. Anesthesiology 73:671–685, 1990

19. Kirklin JK, Blackstone EH, Kirklin JW: Cardiopulmonary bypass: Studies on its damaging effects. Blood Purif 5:168–178, 1987

20. Haeffner-Cavaillon N, Roussellier N, Ponzio O, Carreno MP, Laude M, Carpentier A, Kazatchkine MD: Induction of interleukin-1 production in patients undergoing cardiopulmonary bypass. J Thorac Cardiovasc Surg 98:1100–1106, 1989

21. Gillinov AM, Redmond JM, Winkelstein JA, Zehr KJ, Herskowitz A, Baumgartner WA, Cameron DE. Complement and neutrophil activation during cardiopulmonary bypass: A study in the complement-deficient dog. Ann Thorac Surg 57:345–352, 1994

22. Gillinov AM, De Valeria PA, Winkelstein JA, Wilson I, Curtis WE, Shaw D, Yeh CG, Rudolph AR, Baumgartner WA, Herskowitz A, et al: Complement inhibition with soluble complement receptor type 1 in cardiopulmonary bypass. Ann Thorac Surg 55:619–624, 1993

23. Hirthler M, Simoni J, Dickson M: Elevated levels of endotoxin, oxygen-derived free radicals, and cytokines during extracorporeal membrane oxygenation. J Pediatr Surg 27:1199–1202, 1992

24. Casey LC: Role of cytokines in the pathogenesis of cardiopulmonary-induced multisystem organ failure. Ann Thorac Surg 56:S92–S96, 1993

25. Bellomo R, Tipping P, Boyce N: Continuous veno-venous hemofiltration with dialysis removes cytokines from the circulation of septic patients. Crit Care Med 21:522–526, 1993

26. Storck M, Hartl WH, Zimmerer E, Inthorn D: Comparison of pump-driven and spontaneous haemofiltration in postoperative acute renal failure. Lancet 337:452–455, 1991

27. Journois D, Chanu D, Safran D: Pump-driven haemofiltration. Lancet 337: 985, 1991

28. Barrera P, Janssen EM, Demacker PN, Wetzels JF, van der Meer JW: Removal of interleukin-1 beta and tumor necrosis factor from human plasma by in vitro dialysis with polyacrylonitrile membranes. Lymphokine Cytokine Res 11:99–104, 1992

29. Haeffner-Cavaillon N, Cavaillon JM, Ciancioni C, Bacle F, Delons S, Kazatchkine MD: In vivo induction of interleukin-1 during hemodialysis. Kidney Int 35:1212–1218, 1989

30. Laude-Sharp M, Caroff M, Simard L, Pusineri C, Kazatchkine MD, Haeffner-Cavaillon N: Induction of IL-1 during hemodialysis: Transmembrane passage of intact endotoxins. Kidney Int 38:1089–1094, 1990

31. Cavaillon JM, Fitting C, Haeffner-Cavaillon N: Recombinant C5a enhances interleukin-1 and tumor necrosis factor release by lipopolysaccharide-stimulated monocytes and macrophages. Eur J Immunol 20:253–257, 1990

32. Neote K, Darbonne W, Ogez J, Horuk R, Schall TJ: Identification of a promiscuous inflammatory peptide receptor on the surface of red blood cells. J Biol Chem 268:12247–12249, 1993

33. Hopeck JM, Lane RS, Schroeder JW: Oxygenator volume control by parallel ultrafiltration to remove plasma water. Extracorporeal Tech 13: 267–271, 1981

34. den Hollander JM, Hennis PJ, Burm AG, Vletter AA, Bovill JG: Pharmacokinetics of alfentanil before and after cardiopulmonary bypass in pediatric patients undergoing cardiac surgery: Part I. J Cardiothorac Vasc Anesth 6:308–312, 1992

35. Hynynen M, Hynninen M, Soini H, Neuvonen PJ, Heinonen J: Plasma concentration and protein binding of alfentanil during high-dose infusion for cardiac surgery. Br J Anaesth 72:571–576, 1994

36. Gombotz H, Vukovitch TH, Fall A, et al: Aprotinin levels in patients with hemofiltration during EEC (abstr). 14th SCA meeting, Boston, May 3–6, 1992

Frederick A. Burrows
Francis X. McGowan, Jr.

Neurodevelopmental Consequences of Cardiac Surgery for Congenital Heart Disease

5

Neurological deficits remain the most dreaded of complications after cardiac surgery. In the past, analysis of outcomes after cardiac surgery for complex congenital heart lesions (CHD) have concentrated on survival. However, surgical mortality of neonates, infants, and children undergoing repair of CHD has undergone dramatic reduction in the last 10 years. The estimated in-hospital death rate has been reported to be as low as 3.0 (2.1 to 4.3).[1] With improvement in survival statistics has come the recognition of a significant incidence of adverse neurological sequelae.

Although abnormalities of the central nervous system may be a function of coexisting cerebral abnormalities[2,3] or acquired events unrelated to surgical management,[4] insults to the central nervous system appear to occur most frequently during or immediately after cardiac surgery. Recent reports suggest that transient or permanent neuropsychiatric injury may occur in as many as 25% of all infants undergoing hypothermic cardiopulmonary bypass (CPB) with or without deep hypothermic circulatory arrest (DHCA).[5] In complex palliative procedures, the reported incidence of neuropsychiatric impairment has been much higher. Glauser et al.[6] has reported an incidence of 45% in patients undergoing repair of hypoplastic left heart syndrome. This high incidence of neuropsychiatric impairment serves as a focus for research into the etiology and prevention of cerebral injury during CPB.

Perioperative Management of the Patient with Congenital Heart Disease, edited by William J. Greeley. Williams & Wilkins, Baltimore © 1996.

MECHANISMS OF NEUROLOGICAL INJURY

There are three primary mechanisms of neurological injury during CPB. Mechanical injury occurs from emboli that are the result of trauma to diseased blood vessels or of the intracardiac entrapment of air or particles after cardiac procedures. Microemboli are produced by interactions between blood and the myriad artificial surfaces present in the CPB circuit. Transcranial Doppler monitoring of blood flow suggests that cerebral microemboli occur in all patients undergoing CPB.[6a]

The second type of injury results from alterations in blood flow and distribution, leading to a change in pressure-flow autoregulation, cellular metabolism, and the response to reperfusion.[7-11] Cardiopulmonary bypass may produce nonphysiological flow because of the abnormal site of return of oxygenated blood from the pump, the lack of pulsatile flow from most pumps, the need for low-flow CPB or circulatory arrest to facilitate surgical repair, and other factors that affect blood flow, such as blood pH and temperature.

Finally, environmental, pharmacological, and patient-related factors influence the postoperative psychological state of surgical patients. The additive effects of sleep deprivation, neuroleptic drugs, anxiety, pain, and isolation from family have long been recognized as important determinants of psychological well-being. Extremes of age, cyanosis,[12] cerebrovascular atherosclerosis, and cardiac disease predispose patients to neurological injury.

The risk of neurological injury differs, depending on the particular support technique used. DHCA arrest, defined as the cessation of all blood flow in the body, serves as the worst-case scenario for global neurological ischemia. This procedure has been used routinely in children in the repair of congenital cardiac defects. Hypothermia is the current mainstay of cerebral protection. Hypothermia not only decreases cerebral metabolism but also increases tissue content of high-energy phosphates and intracellular pH, both of which improve the tolerance of ischemia. The alteration of blood pH, the prevention of hyperglycemia, the use of drugs that decrease cerebral metabolism, and the administration of calcium and β-blockers, N-methyl-D-aspartic acid receptor antagonists, steroids, and free-radical scavengers have all been proposed as beneficial.[13-15] The metabolic basis of neurological injury of the brain during CPB will be discussed in greater detail after the discussion of the existing clinical studies.

DIFFERENCES IN PEDIATRIC CPB

Although subtle neurological injury is not uncommon in adult patients undergoing CPB, the management and physiological impact of

CPB in adults is very different from that in pediatric patients, and the etiology of the cerebral injury may be quite different. During hypothermic CPB there are multiple variables that might influence the risk of cerebral injury (Table 5–1). It is likely that there is interaction between these various elements, such that the etiology of cerebral injury after CPB is multifactorial. Compared with the adult patient, pediatric patients undergo biological extremes, including deep hypothermia (15 to 20°C), hemodilution (three- to fourfold dilution of circulating blood volume), low perfusion pressures (20 to 30 mm Hg), wide variation in pump flow rates (ranging from highs of 200 ml/kg/min to DHCA), and wide-ranging blood-gas management. These unphysiological parameters significantly alter cerebral regulatory function and probably affect neurological outcome. In addition to these prominent changes, subtle variations in glucose supplementation, cannula placement, presence of aortopulmonary collaterals, patient age, and brain mass may also affect cerebral preservation during CPB. Because of these differences in CPB management when compared to those of adult patients, extrapolation of the adult experience on the effects of bypass on the central nervous system to the pediatric patient must be made cautiously. Certain of these perfusion variables have been examined in relation to their influence on subsequent neurodevelopment.

PERFUSION VARIABLES

Rate and Duration of Core Cooling

Cerebral protection by hypothermia is based on the premise that there is a significant fall in cerebral metabolism and oxygen consumption that is related to cerebral temperature. Recent studies suggest that hypothermia alone can account for the majority of the protection ob-

TABLE 5–1.   PERFUSION VARIABLES WITH POTENTIAL FOR PRODUCING NEUROLOGICAL INJURY

Duration of CPB
Duration and rate of core cooling
Acid-base management during core cooling
Duration of circulatory arrest
Type of oxygenator
Arterial filtration
Depth of hypothermia
Management of hematocrit
Management of anticoagulation
Management of serum glucose

served during DHCA.[9] Other variables, such as anesthetic agents, provide much smaller contributions to cerebral protection, once deep hypothermic temperatures (15 to 20°C) are reached.[16]

Cerebral protection afforded by core cooling on CPB assumes that homogenous cooling of all regions of the brain occurs. Recent studies have suggested that this may not be so. Kern et al. measured the venous oxygen saturations of effluent blood from the jugular venous bulb during cooling CPB (Fig. 5–1). However, despite an adequate tympanic temperature, considerable variation in saturations were seen despite equal duration of cooling. A cooling duration of approximately 18 minutes was necessary to ensure adequate suppression of metabolic activity, as measured by jugular venous oxygen saturations.[17] Other workers[18] have demonstrated an increase in the temperature of jugular venous effluent blood in the presence of stable tympanic and aortic inflow temperature when low-flow CPB is established (Fig. 5–2). As such, standard monitoring of tympanic temperatures may not identify all patients with inadequately cooled brains

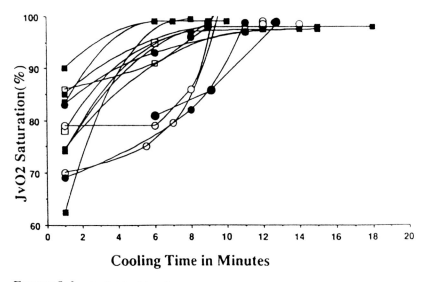

Cooling Time in Minutes

FIGURE 5–1. Individual jugular venous oxygen (JvO_2) saturation data are plotted vs cooling time for CPB samples. For each individual patient, the bypass measurements of JvO_2 saturation are extrapolated to a point of 100% jugular venous saturation. Patients demonstrating jugular venous desaturation could not be identified clinically. Low JvO_2 saturations suggest higher levels of cerebral metabolism and cerebral uptake of oxygen. In the presence of deep hypothermic CPB and stable anesthetic levels, the most likely cause of a low JvO_2 saturation is inadequate cerebral cooling. (Reproduced with permission from Kern FH, et al. Ann Thorac Surg 54:749–754, 1992)

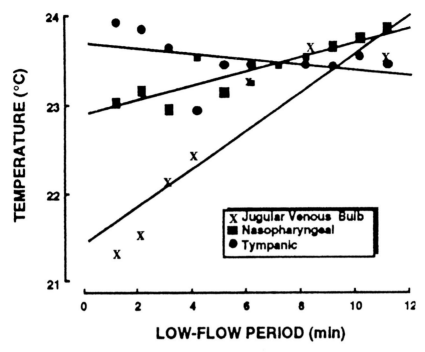

FIGURE 5–2. Linear regression analysis and lines of best fit were used to represent the change in jugular venous bulb, nasopharyngeal and tympanic temperatures when low-flow cardiopulmonary bypass was instituted and aortic inflow temperature was held constant. While aortic, nasopharyngeal, and tympanic temperatures were constant, jugular venous bulb temperature increased. The clinical implication is that currently used temperature monitoring sites may not reflect the actual brain temperature and inadequate cerebral cooling may be present. (Reproduced with permission from Foster JMT, et al. Anesthesiology 79:A1144, 1993.)

and continuing cerebral metabolism. Inhomogeneity of cerebral cooling in some patients may be related to the position of the aortic cannula, age, or biological variability. Institutional variability in the rate of core cooling, such as rapid or more gradual cooling, may also result in different degrees of homogeneity of cerebral cooling.[19] Adjunctive therapies of cerebral cooling such as topical cooling of the head with ice have also been reported to be effective.[20]

To evaluate the influence of core cooling on CPB on subsequent neurodevelopment, Bellinger and colleagues[21] retrospectively reviewed 28 neonates and infants who underwent the arterial switch operation for transposition of the great arteries between 1983 and 1988. The surgical procedure was performed, using DHCA (64.5 ± 9.8 min). The cooling period entailed maintaining hypothermic temperatures while continuing full CPB flow (150 ml/kg/min). Patients were tested with age-appropriated developmental tests, age-normed to have a mean score of 100 ± 16.

The intraoperative variable most strongly associated with cognitive development was the duration of core cooling before DHCA. The relationship was curvilinear, with the strongest association in the group with shorter cooling times (11 to 18 min). Within this rate of core cooling an increase of 5 minutes was associated with a 26-point increase in development score (Figs. 5–3 to 5–5). It was speculated that the shorter period of cooling before DHCA resulted in inhomogeneous cooling with the brain and areas in which metabolism had not slowed adequately remaining vulnerable to damage during DHCA. Patients cooled for more prolonged periods on CPB (20 to 39 min) showed a trend toward worse developmental outcome with longer cooling times, although this trend did not reach statistical significance. It is speculated that the potential benefits of prolonged core cooling begin to be offset by the known sources of brain injury related to the length of CPB, such as microembolic events.

Acid-Base Management During Core Cooling

Arterial pH and P_{CO_2} play an important role in regulating cerebral blood flow both physiologically and during CPB. However, the optimal strategy for management of pH and P_{CO_2} during profound hypothermia, with or without DHCA, is controversial.[22-28] Both the pH-stat and α-stat strategies have theoretical disadvantages. The pH-stat strategy may result in loss of autoregulation. By increasing cerebral blood flow beyond metabolic requirements, the pH-stat strategy may lead to an increased potential for cerebral microembolization, increased brain edema, and intracranial hypertension.[25] In contrast, the α-stat strategy results in less cerebral blood flow, as well as a shift to the left of the oxyhemoglobin dissociation curve; in the context of low perfusion pressures, flows, and temperatures, cerebral perfusion under α-stat strategy could be inadequate to meet metabolic needs and perhaps inadequate to allow homogeneous cooling before DHCA.

It is unclear as to whether developmental outcome in pediatric patients is affected by the particular pH strategy used. To attempt to answer this question, Jonas et al. retrospectively reviewed 16 patients between the ages of 2 and 154 days (median, 32 days), with a diagnosis of transposition of the great arteries and intact ventricular septum who underwent repair by the Senning procedure during the period between 1983 and 1988.[29] They collected information on many aspects of perfusion, including lowest P_{CO_2} during core cooling, du-

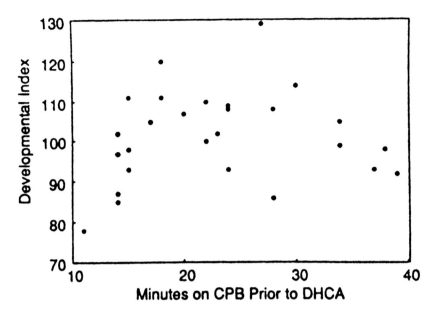

FIGURE 5-3. Scatterplot of core cooling (minutes of CPB before DHCA) and developmental index. (Reproduced with permission from Bellinger DC, et al. Pediatrics 87:705–707, 1991)

ration of core cooling, and duration of circulatory arrest. The pH strategy was changed from pH-stat to α-stat in 1985, resulting in a wide range of pH values and Pco_2 tension (34 to 76 mm Hg) during the study period. All patients had rapid core cooling to a mean ($\pm$SD) rectal temperature of 19.8 $\pm$ 2.7°C and a tympanic temperature of 16.6 $\pm$ 3.0°C. The mean duration of core cooling was 14.5 $\pm$ 6.2 minutes, DHCA duration was 43.4 $\pm$ 6.6 minutes, and total CPB plus DHCA time was 89.7 $\pm$ 12.7 minutes. Development was assessed at a median age of 48.0 (11 to 19) months with the Bayley Scales[30] of Infant Development (n = 4, children younger than 30 mo) or the McCarthy Scales[31] of Children's Abilities (n = 12, children older than 30 mo). Lower Pco_2 (α-stat) before the onset of DHCA was associated with worse developmental outcome. Over the range of approximately 30 to 80 mm HG developmental score increased 8.8 points for every 10 mm Hg increase in Pco_2. This relationship remained highly significant when controlled for sociodemographic and intraoperative variables, including core cooling time, duration of DHCA, and total elapsed time.

The improved cognitive result obtained with the pH-stat strategy may be related to the increased cerebral blood flow[25] that might result

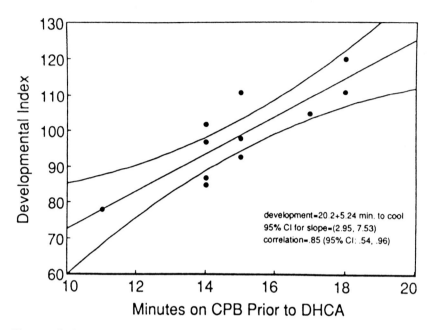

FIGURE 5-4. Scatterplot of core cooling (minutes of CPB before DHCA) and developmental index for infants with "short" periods of core cooling (<20 min). The best-fit regression line and 95% confidence interval (CI) are shown. (Reproduced with permission from Bellinger DC, et al. Pediatrics, 87:701–705, 1991)

in more homogeneous brain cooling. In addition, the relative acidosis of the pH-stat strategy counteracts the leftward shift in the oxyhemoglobin dissociation curve, which results from the hypothermia. This effect may be important when rapid core cooling is used, particularly in the early phases of cooling, when relatively cool blood may be unable to deliver sufficient oxygen to as-yet warm areas of the brain.

Deep Hypothermic Circulatory Arrest

Early Postoperative Sequelae of Circulatory Arrest

The immature brain has a lower threshold to seizures, and their frequency in the neonatal and infant period is higher than at any other stage of life.[32] The recent trend toward early neonatal repair of complex congenital cardiac lesions thus potentially shifts this population toward higher risk. It is not surprising, therefore, that seizures are the

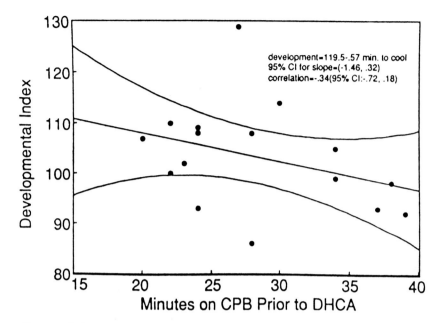

FIGURE 5–5. Scatterplot of core cooling (minutes of CPB before DHCA) and developmental index for infants with "long" periods of core cooling (≥20 min). The best-fit regression line and 95% confidence interval (CI) are shown. (Reproduced with permission from Bellinger DC, et al. Pediatrics 87:701–707, 1991)

most frequently observed neurological consequence of cardiac surgery with the use of DHCA, with a reported incidence of 4 to 25%, depending on the length of the circulatory arrest period.[7] Both focal and generalized seizures have been described, usually occurring on the first through fourth postoperative days.

There is, however, no universally accepted definition of seizure activity in the neonate and young infant. The differences between normal patterns of behavior, abnormal but nonictal behavior, and true seizure activity are less distinct in the newborn than at any other age[32] and often present a diagnostic challenge. Of the different clinical patterns described (i.e., clonic, tonic, myoclonic and "subtle" seizures),[33] it is the motor automatisms and autonomic paroxysms of "subtle" seizures that are the most difficult to distinguish from the normal movements of the young infant or the abnormal nonictal behavior patterns of the encephalopathic or sedated infant.[34,35] The use of long-term videoelectroencephalography has been increasingly used in the detection of seizures in children. This technology allows simultaneous 15-16 channel recordings to be compared with visual examination of the patient and/or various physiological monitoring tracings in patients after cardiac surgery. Studies using such recordings in newborns not having undergone cardiac surgery have shown a high incidence of "silent" electrocortical ictal activity that was not manifest clinically.[7,36] These "electroencephalogram (EEG) seizures" occur most often in the setting of stupor or coma, after the onset of anticonvulsant therapy, and in pharmacologically paralyzed infants.

The true incidence of postoperative seizures is, therefore, a complex issue. The incidence of clinical seizures may be overestimated, due to the difficulties in distinguishing between normal and abnormal movements in neonates and young infants. Conversely, the incidence may be underestimated, in part, because the frequent use of paralytic or sedative agents (e.g., benzodiazepines) in the early postoperative period obscures the clinical manifestations of seizure activity.

Although the long-term prognosis after hypoxic-ischemic seizures in the (normothermic) neonate may be guarded, the long-term significance of seizures occurring after hypothermic bypass with circulatory arrest is unknown. The most powerful criteria for predicting outcome in noncardiac patients suffering neonatal and early infantile seizures are the underlying etiology of the seizure and the background features of the interictal electroencephalograph. These criteria are not easily applied to the neonate or infant with seizures after cardiac surgery as the exact etiological mechanisms are not always clear. Although any of the usual metabolic, vascular, and infectious etiologies may underlie these seizures, there appears to be a group of transient ictal events peculiar to this population. These seizures appear to have several distinguishing features. They tend to be present in the second 24 hours after surgery, may be either generalized or focal clinical events, and are easily controlled with anticonvulsants. A largely anecdotal study suggested no long-term neurological morbidity, an increased risk for late seizures or the need for chronic anticonvulsant therapy in a small group of patients who had clinically "unexplained" seizures after cardiac surgery in infancy.[37] The lack of prospectively gathered data and a "normative" database in this population of infants for electroencephalography also compromises, at this point, the use of intraoperative or postoperative recordings in long-term prognostication.

A more recent study addresses this question in a more well-controlled, prospective fashion. The Boston Circulatory Arrest Study (BCAS) examined the developmental and neurological sequelae of 171 neonates and infants with D-transposition of the great arteries (with or without a ventricular septal defect), who underwent an arterial switch operation and were randomly assigned to a method of support consisting predominantly of circulatory arrest or a method consisting predominantly of low-flow bypass. In the immediate postoperative period, patients assigned to the circulatory arrest group demonstrated a tendency to a higher risk of clinical seizures and ictal activity on continuous EEG monitoring during the first 48 hours after surgery (Fig. 5–6). They also demonstrated a longer recovery time to the first reappearance of EEG activity and a greater release of the brain isoenzyme of creatine kinase.[7]

Choreoathetosis

The incidence of choreoathetosis has been estimated to be between 1 and 12%. Although commonly believed to arise in patients undergoing DHCA,[38] the condition has been noted to occur in infants and children undergoing CPB and hypothermia without circulatory arrest.[39] Numerous events during CPB or DHCA have been suggested as etiologies, including hyperglycemia,[40] uneven cooling,[41] the noreflow phenomenon,[42,43] dopaminergic neurotransmitter alterations,[44] and cerebral excitatory amino acid neurotoxicity.[38] No single etiology has been universally accepted, nor have a constant set of risk factors been identified. Two degrees of severity of choreoathetosis have been identified: a mild, transient form that resolves completely within 6

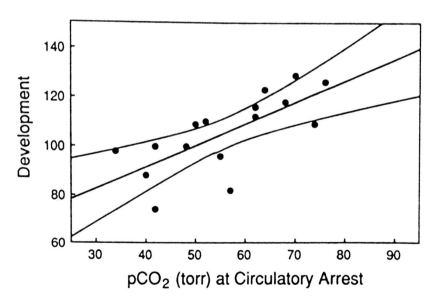

FIGURE 5–6. Association between postoperative cognitive function and arterial PCO2 (as measured at 37°C) before deep hypothermic circulatory arrest. ($r = .71$, $P = .002$). (Reproduced with permission from Jonas RA, et al. J Thorac Cardiovasc Surg 106:362–368, 1993)

months and a severe, persistent form in which movements continued.[45] They suggested that choreoathetosis may be an age-related phenomenon, with the most vulnerable period starting at 6 to 9 months
and ending after 5 to 6 years. Younger patients (<8 mo), when affected, appear to have a milder form of choreoathetosis and, generally,
a better overall prognosis for recovery from the movement disorder.
In contrast, the development of severe choreoathetosis in older patients (>6 mo) carries a significantly worse prognosis. The mortality
rate in patients with the persistent form of the syndrome, in their
study, was 36%. In addition to age beyond infancy, other factors associated with the development of severe choreoathetosis included the
presence of cyanotic heart disease with systemic to pulmonary collaterals and, possibly, the duration of the cooling period. They speculated
that the presence of systemic-to-pulmonary collaterals may have
served as a cerebral steal on CPB, slowing the normal rate of cerebral
cooling and suggested that the optimal time for cerebral cooling on
CPB in these patients may be longer than that normally accepted.[45]

Late Postoperative Sequelae of Circulatory Arrest

Psychological and intellectual development of children after cardiac
surgery, using DHCA, has been addressed in a number of studies, but
results have been conflicting. Several studies have suggested that the
duration of circulatory arrest has little or no important influence on
later development, whereas others caution against its use. Many studies contend that patient-related variables (such as low birth weight,
preoperative illness, preexisting neurological abnormalities, age at operation, duration of cyanosis, socioeconomic status, and other factors)
play a more significant role in later development than the intraoperative effects of CPB and DHCA. Thus, the identification of an adequate
control is crucial in determining the effects of DHCA on later development.

Blackwood et al.[46] tested 36 children with both cyanotic and acyanotic CHD before and 4 to 29 months after surgery, using the patients
as their own controls. Circulatory arrest was used in 26 of 36 patients.
Their results suggested no relationship between circulatory arrest and
either the duration of DHCA or age at operation on developmental
quotient. Higher socioeconomic status was significantly positively correlated with later outcome.

Clarkson and colleagues[47] studied 72 children with heterogeneous
forms of CHD repaired at 0.2 to 26 months of age, using DHCA. Follow-up testing was performed 29 to 84 months after surgery. Test
results were compared to those of a matched group of preschool

children randomly selected from a sequential group of children born at one hospital. The results suggested no relationship between intelligence quotient and either duration of circulatory arrest, age at operation, or race. Low birth weight, preoperative neurological abnormalities, and low socioeconomic status impacted negatively on later outcome.

Wells et al.[48] studied 31 patients undergoing repair of both cyanotic and acyanotic lesions, using circulatory arrest. Three control groups were used: 19 children undergoing repair, by means of moderate hypothermic bypass without DHCA; 16 siblings of the study patients; and 14 siblings of the patients undergoing repair without DHCA. The mean intelligence quotient of the patient managed with arrest was 91 ± 4 SE, lower than each comparison group (moderate hypothermia, 102 ± 5.2; siblings of the study patients, 106 ± 4.1; siblings of nonarrested patients, 96 ± 5.9). The difference between the intelligence of the patients repaired with DHCA and their siblings, particularly in the verbal subtests, was linearly related to the duration of DHCA. The intelligence quotient of patients repaired without DHCA was comparable to that of their siblings. Age at operation or age at testing were not related to later outcome.

In addition to generalized development delay and focal neurological findings, more specific long-term sequelae after CPB and DHCA have been reported. Delays in the use of expressive language and verbal reasoning are reported with fairly high frequency,[21,46,48–50] as are inattentiveness and "hyperactivity."[49,50] Gross and fine motor delays are also common findings.[46,49]

The BCAS recently completed their 1-year postsurgery follow-up.[51] They found that patients in the DHCA group demonstrated a lower mean score on the Psychomotor Development Index of the Bayley Scale of Infant Development, as compared to those assigned to low-flow bypass (Fig. 5–7). The score on the Psychomotor Development Index was inversely related to the duration of circulatory arrest. The risk of neurological abnormalities increased with the duration of circulatory arrest (Fig. 5–8). The method of support was not associated with the prevalence of abnormalities on magnetic resonance imaging (MRI) scans of the brain, scores on the Mental Development Index of the Bayley Scale, or scores on a test of visual recognition memory. However, perioperative EEG seizure activity was associated with lower scores on the Psychomotor Development Index and an increased likelihood of abnormalities on MRI scans of the brain (Fig. 5–9).

In summary, the developmental and neurological status of children receiving a management strategy consisting predominantly of DHCA as a method of supporting vital organs during surgery for

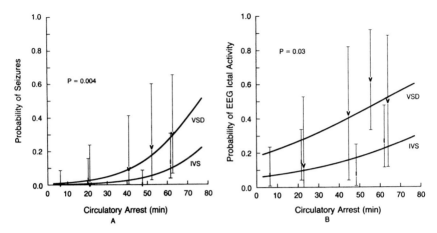

FIGURE 5-7. Estimated probabilities of definite seizures in the first week after surgery (A) and of ictal activity on continuous video EEG in the first 48 hours after surgery (B), as a function of the duration of total circulatory arrest. Logistic-regression curves are shown for infants with an intact ventricular septum (IVS) and for those with a ventricular septal defect (VSD). In addition, point estimates and exact 95% confidence intervals for outcome probabilities are plotted for the mean of each quartile of duration of circulatory arrest (I and V for the respective groups). The P values shown were calculated by logistic regression for the effect of the duration of circulatory arrest on outcome, with adjustment for diagnosis. (Reproduced with permission from Newburger JW, et al. N Engl J Med 329:1057–1064, 1993)

repair of CHD appears to be worse than that of children who are managed predominantly with low-flow CPB. Further assessments of such children at older ages are necessary to clarify whether these findings predict clinically important differences in academic function.

Management of Glucose

Clinical and laboratory studies have implicated hyperglycemia as an exacerbating factor in the outcome of normothermic cerebral ischemia in the mature adult brain.[52–55] Avoidance of glucose administration has been recommended in adults undergoing cardiac surgery, even those not undergoing planned cerebral ischemia.[56,57] In children undergoing corrective cardiac surgery, the effects of glucose on neurological outcome are less clear.[58] The BCAS has examined the relationship of intraoperative serum glucose to indices of potential neurological damage in the perioperative period.[59] They were unable to correlate blood glucose levels before DHCA or low-flow CPB with any indices

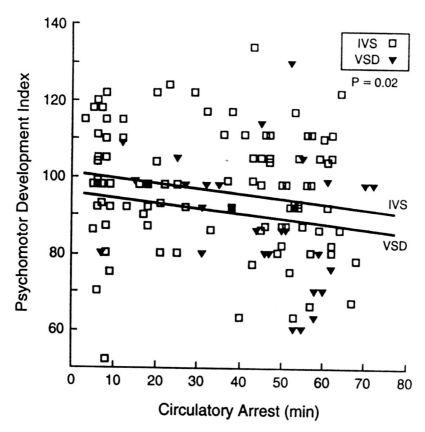

FIGURE 5–8. Score on the Psychomotor Development Index at 1 year as a function of the duration of total circulatory arrest. Regression lines are shown for children with an intact ventricular septum (*IVS*) and those with a ventricular septal defect (*VSD*). The *P* value shown was calculated by linear regression for the effect of duration of total circulatory arrest on the score on the Psychomotor Development Index, with adjustment for diagnosis. (Reproduced with permission from Bellinger DC, et al. N Engl J Med 332:549–555, 1995)

of poor neurological outcome, except for a weak ($r = .22$) correlation between high glucose levels immediately before DHCA and creatine kinase (CK) (brain) release (Fig. 5–10). However, blood glucose levels, measured at multiple periods during the reperfusion period after DHCA, did not correlate with postoperative CK-BB release into serum. Similarly, no positive association was demonstrated between hyperglycemia at any time during the operation and neurological dysfunction as measured by EEG and clinical parameters. What was demonstrated was an association between blood glucose during reperfusion and better outcome, as judged by means of these same

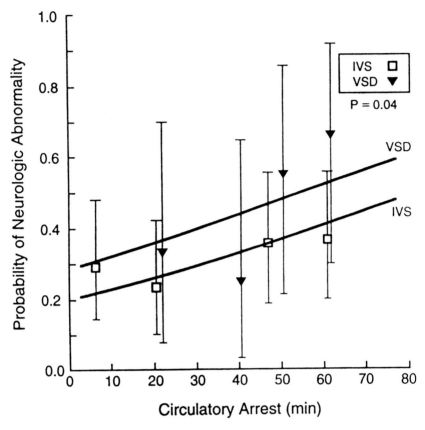

FIGURE 5-9. Estimated probability for a possible or definite neurological abnormality at 1 year of age as a function of the duration of total circulatory arrest. Logistic-regression lines are shown for children with an intact ventricular septum (IVS) and those with a ventricular septal defect (VSD). Point estimates and exact 95% confidence intervals for outcome probabilities are plotted for the means of each quartile for the duration of circulatory arrest. The *P* value was calculated by logistic regression for the effect of the duration of circulatory arrest on the neurologic outcome, with adjustment for diagnosis. (Reproduced with permission from Bellinger DC, et al. N Engl J Med 332:549–555, 1995)

parameters (Fig. 5–11). This is in agreement with the results of experimental studies in immature animals, which suggest that preischemic hyperglycemia does not exacerbate ischemic damage in the immature brain and that hyperglycemia on reperfusion may ameliorate such damage.[60–65] The BCAS determined that "normal" blood glucose levels were associated with poorer neurological outcome and hyperglycemic levels were associated with better outcome. These associations were particularly strong in the arrest group, which was subjected to the

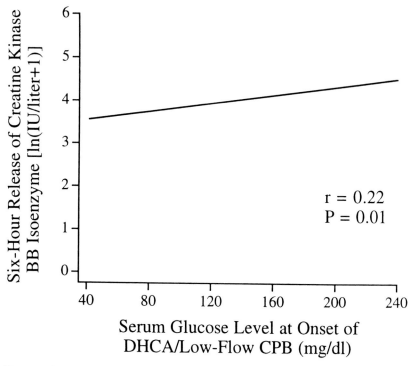

FIGURE 5–10. Six-hour release of creatine kinase BB isoenzyme (CK-BB) as a function of serum glucose level at the onset of circulatory arrest or low-flow CPB. The correlation coefficient measures the strength of the linear relationship between CK-BB and glucose level and does not adjust for diagnosis. Six-hour release of CK-BB is expressed as the natural logarithm of the integrated measurement plus 1. (Courtesy of Dr. P. R. Hickey)

longest duration of DHCA. The authors speculate that in the immature brain, a cellular metabolic picture more characteristic of substrate deficiency than oxygen deficiency results from ischemia and that "normal" glucose levels during the reperfusion period after cerebral ischemia in infants may be insufficient for complete cerebral recovery.

METHODOLOGICAL LIMITATIONS

Many of these studies must be interpreted cautiously. Some are complicated by methodological flaws. Such flaws include small sample sizes with limited statistical power; heterogeneous congenital lesions; different methods of achieving hypothermic conditions (e.g., surface vs core cooling); different ages at operation, testing, and follow-up;

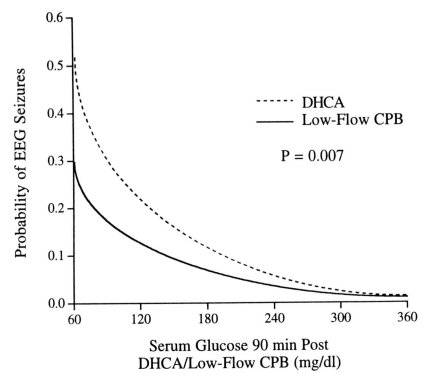

FIGURE 5-11. Estimated probability of EEG seizures as a function of the serum glucose level 90 minutes after the end of circulatory arrest or low-flow bypass. Logistic regression curves are shown for infants assigned to the predominant DHCA group and for those assigned to the predominant low-flow bypass group (LF). The *P* value was calculated by logistic regression for the effect of glucose level on the probability of EEG seizures, adjusting for treatment group and diagnosis. (Courtesy of Dr. P. R. Hickey)

different testing modalities; failure to identify an adequate "control" group with appropriate identification of social class, birth order, and perinatal events; inadequate adjustment for and/or investigation of preexisting lesions in the central nervous system.

Prospective evaluations by neurologists have consistently found a higher incidence of neurological morbidity, compared with the findings of cardiologists or cardiac surgeons.[5] Additionally, most long-term studies focus on intelligence or development quotients, with a broad definition of normalcy and with only limited attempts to differentiate the potential impact of the independent variables on important component skills (e.g., attention, visual-motor integration, expressive and receptive language). Extrapolation of laboratory-based investigations to clinically relevant measures of outcome has rarely been performed. There are inherent difficulties in the developmental assessment of young children, which may limit the inferences one may make with regard to long-term function. In the BCAS, in particular, the relative deficits of the children assigned to the predominantly DHCA group were most prominent in the domain of motor function, but assessments at older ages may reveal treatment effects in other domains, such as language or visual-motor integration, that are not easily tested in very young children.

These preliminary clinical studies, nonetheless, form the basis of our understanding of the pathophysiology of injury to the central nervous system during cardiac surgery and provide the impetus for further investigations. The remainder of this chapter will discuss laboratory experience with the immature nervous system and etiologies of cerebral injury in children with CHD.

NEURODEVELOPMENTAL TASKS OF THE IMMATURE CENTRAL NERVOUS SYSTEM

Human brain development occurs in a highly ordered and coordinated progression of events. After the initial stages of neuroblast and neural tube formation, first and second trimester brain development is highlighted by multiplication and migration of both neuronal and glial cells in the germinal matrix region adjacent to the lateral ventricle and striatum[66]; much of the forebrain and cerebral cortex are formed during this time. Toward the end of gestation, significant glial multiplication and myelinization take place. Glial development provides pathways for neurons migrating outward to destinations in the cerebral cortex and elsewhere. Glia also synthesize myelin and create a framework for brain growth and organization. Glial development continues from the first trimester through the first year of life, whereas neuronal multiplication in the brain is essentially complete at term. The brain grows exponentially during the first 2 to 3 postnatal years, weighing approximately 350 gm at birth, 900 gm at 1 year, and 1400 gm in the adult.[67] The bulk of this growth is due to glial expansion, progressive myelinization, axonal development, neuronal differentiation, dendritic development, and synaptogenesis.

Neuronal multiplication in the fetus may occur at a peak rate of 250,000 neurons/minutes, resulting in a final complement of approximately 100 billion neurons.[68] Nonetheless, glial cells eventually outnumber neurons by about 10 to 1. It has become clear that glia and neurons interact in a bidirectional manner and that these interactions influence neuronal development, maturation, and viability and are also critical for such processes as long-term potentiation, memory, and cytotoxicity.

The regulation of this rapid expansion and development must be coordinated and precise. It is under the control of genetic, environmental, local cellular, humoral, neurotransmitter, and trophic factors. As mentioned previously, neuronal migration takes place along glial paths, with later-developing neurons that are migrating to cortical layers traveling past early developing ones that remain situated in deeper layers close to the germinal matrix.[69] Factors that regulate neuronal migration are not known, but evidence of control by genetic programming, neurotransmitters, excitatory amino acids, and neural cellular adhesion molecules has been presented.[69–71] Likewise, the factors that contribute to axonal growth and localization of specific target cells are poorly understood but are also felt to be under the influence of local cell-to-cell molecular communication, trophic factors, excitatory amino acids, neurotransmitters, and external stimuli.

There appears to be significant interplay between axonal development, dendritic branching, and synapse formation. Dendrite growth proceeds essentially in parallel with axonal ingrowth and synaptogenesis and is also influenced by intrinsic neuronal factors. Innervation and synapse activity are also critical to dendritic development. Synaptogenesis and synapse remodeling also require the cooperation of trophic factors, excitatory amino acids, neurotransmitters, and localization of appropriate target cells. This last process may be influenced by specific membrane receptors, including those linked to glutamate and gamma-aminobutyric acid (GABA).

However, all is not growth and expansion. Neuronal and synaptic deletion are critical to normal brain development as well. Depending on the brain region, as many as approximately 50% of the connections formed during the first 1 to 2 years of life will be absent by ages 10 to 20. The choice of synapses to be maintained is influenced by a number of factors, including genetic program, excitatory amino acids (see below), and neuronal activity produced by external stimuli.[70,72] Trophic substances such as nerve growth factor (NGF) produced by specific target cells stimulate the growth and development of NGF-dependent neurons; in its absence, they die.[73] Other such trophic and inhibitory substances include neurotransmitters and other types of NGFs.

Finally, the recently described phenomenon of apoptosis, or programmed cell death, is likely to contribute to deletion of specific neurons during normal brain development.[74,75] As noted above, neural proliferation and development is controlled by internal cell programming, neuronal activity, and responses to external growth factors and regulatory stimuli. These responses are mediated through a variety of intracellular signal transduction cascades that result in altered gene expression and protein synthesis. Apoptosis can be viewed as an opposing mechanism, activated by hormonal and other factors, as well as by growth factor deprivation, that triggers a novel genetic program, resulting in cell death. Apoptosis was initially described in the nematode *C. elegans*, where 118 of a total of 302 neurons die in a highly specific, programmed fashion that is under the control of several gene products.[76,77] Several genes in mammals (including humans) have been associated with control of apoptosis in normal and tumor cells, and evidence for its participation in cell death from stroke and other forms of ischemia-reperfusion injury has been presented.[78,79] Cell death from cytokines, free radicals, and calcium may, in part, involve activation of an apoptotic program.

CPB potentially poses several threats to the orderly progression of brain development in the infant. Metabolical and energetic derangements, leading to cellular dysfunction or death, may result from inadequate oxygen and substrate delivery due to low-flow, circulatory arrest, and anatomical abnormalities. Energetic deprivation and calcium overload can also stimulate amino acid excitotoxicity. Reperfusion activates an additional set of injurious mechanisms, including calcium overload, free radical generation, and influx of inflammatory cells and mediators. Each of these processes can be directly toxic; activate intracellular signaling cascades that promote further membrane damage, radical injury, leukocyte adhesion, and invasion; and lead to both necrotic and apoptotic cell death. These issues will now be discussed in some detail.

Brain Energetics and Metabolism

Lethal cellular injury in the brain is almost always associated with deranged brain energetics.[80] Significant reductions in the high-energy phosphates adenosine triphosphate (ATP) and phosphocreatine (PCr) begin within several minutes of oxygen deprivation, progress over the duration of the insult, and persist into the recovery period. This has been shown in models of perinatal hypoxia-ischemia, as well as in newborn models of hypothermic circulatory arrest.[80,81] The progressive hydrolysis of ATP in ischemic tissue leads to proton accumulation, production of adenosine, and further purine breakdown products that can diffuse out of the cell, as well as increased free radical generation during reperfusion (e.g., xanthine-xanthine oxidase).

During hypoxia or ischemia, anaerobic glycolysis is stimulated by the accumulation of ADP and adenosine monophosphate (AMP) that results from ATP consumption and failure of mitochondrial oxidative metabolism. Glycolysis is much less efficient at generating ATP, as compared to aerobic metabolism (net 2 mol ATP per glucose vs 36 mol ATP per mol glucose). This means that glycolytic flux would have to increase nearly 20-fold to yield equivalent ATP. In fact, maximal glycolytic stimulation can produce only a three- to five-fold increase;[80] furthermore, during ischemia, glycolysis is rapidly inhibited by the accumulation of its end products, namely, lactate, H^+, and NADH.

One major consequence of neuronal ATP depletion is loss of the ability to maintain ionic gradients by means of membrane pumps that use ATP. As a result, Na^+, Cl^-, and H_2O accumulate, leading to loss of electrochemical gradients and to increasing intracellular edema. Calcium will also accumulate, in part due to exchange of intracellular Na^+ for extracellular Ca^{2+} (membrane Na^+/Ca^{2+} exchanger). Increased intracellular Ca^{2+} is believed to be a central mechanism of cellular injury (see below). Failure to rapidly restore high-energy phosphates with reperfusion, as seen in DHCA models,[81] is likely to exacerbate loss of ionic gradients, Na^+ and Ca^{2+} overload, and intracellular edema. ATP depletion and Ca^{2+} accumulation can trigger release of excitatory neurotransmitters such as glutamate. The cause(s) of delayed brain ATP recovery after hypoxic-ischemic injury are unknown but are believed to be due to mitochondrial membrane damage that results in uncoupling of oxidative phosphorylation.[80,82] This may result in part from free radical injury and mitochondrial Ca^{2+} overload.

Only a modicum of information exists about energetic differences in developing brain. The neonatal brain may have higher intrinsic buffering capacity than that of the adult, perhaps increasing its tolerance to intracellular acidosis during hypoxia.[83] Maximum oxidative respiratory capacity and metabolic rates increase in young animals, beginning at about 10 days of age.[84] Similarly, the rate of the creatine kinase reaction, which catalyzes the transfer of high-energy phosphate from PCr to ATP, also increases significantly between 10 to 15 days of age in the rat brain.[85] Whether these changes taking place some time after birth mean that the younger animal is energetically disadvantaged or protected is not clear at present.

Glucose, Lactate, and H^+

It is fairly well-established that hyperglycemis in adult animals and in humans exacerbates injury from normothermic cerebral ischemia.[53-55,62,86] Proposed mechanisms include promotion of lactic acid production and/or increased intracellular acidosis, owing to increased anaerobic glycolytic flux. Increased intracellular osmolarity from glucose loading may be an additional factor. The assumption is that these effects would not occur in the absence of increased circulating glucose concentration.[80] However, another sizeable body of experimental evidence suggests that preischemic hyperglycemia may protect *immature* brain (mainly in rat models) from systemic hypoxia, asphyxia, or hypoxia-ischemia.[60–65,80] Other studies in piglets have shown that preischemic hyperglycemia worsens cerebral injury, whereas elevated glucose levels after ischemia did not affect injury severity.[87] As with adults, hyperglycemia before and during resuscitation in pediatric trauma victims may also be correlated with more severe brain injury.[88]

Care must be taken when extrapolating this experimental evidence to the clinical situation. The majority of the aforementioned investigations used normothermic rat models of hypoxia, usually but not always in conjunction with unilateral or bilateral carotid artery occlusion (hypoxia-ischemia). These models are obviously quite different from those of hypothermic CPB, in which, even if a period of circulatory arrest is used, oxygenation and global brain perfusion are maintained both before and immediately after arrest. Furthermore, the protective effects of hyperglycemia to improve survival or limit histopathological evidence of injury may not be due to brain protection per se but relate mainly to effects that prolong ventilatory effort and improve cardiovascular function in the hyperglycemic, hypoxic-ischemic animal[80]; these benefits are not likely to accrue to the ventilated, perfused patient on cardiopulmonary bypass. However, these results may indirectly underscore the importance of optimizing cardiovascular function (and, hence, CBF) after DHCA.

Other factors suggested as being responsible for glucose-related damage are increased brain lactic acidosis and H^+ accumulation. Although numerous adult studies have shown correlations between blood glucose level, brain lactate concentration, excitatory neurotransmitter release, and brain injury,[88,89] most evidence does not suggest a primary role for damage due to increased lactate accumulation in the neonatal brain.[80,88] Typically, lactate is not found to be significantly elevated in damaged regions of infant brain, suggesting that increased lactate in adult brain may be merely a marker of ischemic injury. Adult brain has markedly increased ability to transport glucose and higher glycolytic flux and, therefore, would be able to generate higher intracellular glucose levels and greater lactate production.[90–92]

In contrast, intracellular acidosis and H^+ accumulation are consistently linked to cellular injury. For example, a close correlation between NADH concentration ($NAD + H^+ \rightarrow NADH$ during oxygen debt) and neuropathological outcome has been observed.[93] Intracellular acidosis can promote efflux of charged high-energy phosphate compounds, inactivate enzymes and other proteins, inhibit glycolysis, and cause release of Ca^{2+} from intracellular stores. DNA fragmentation may be enhanced by a H^+-dependent endonuclease, which may be a link between intracellular acidosis and apoptosis.[94] Protons cause the release of iron from iron-binding proteins, thereby increasing iron-catalyzed free radical production.[95] The production of toxic hydroxyl ($\cdot OH^-$) radicals from peroxynitrite formed by the reaction of nitric oxide ($NO\cdot$) with superoxide ($\cdot O_2^-$) is theoretically enhanced by H^+.[96]

However, other lines of evidence suggest that acidosis can have protective effects. Normo- or hypercapnic mature rats had less severe hypoxic-ischemic brain damage than equivalent subjects ventilated to hypocapnia.[97] Increased pCO_2 may increase tissue pO_2 by decreasing the affinity of hemoglobin for O_2 and may also preserve cardiovascular function. More important to the bypass setting, hypercapnia has been shown to decrease cerebral metabolic rate, energy use, glycolytic flux, and lactate production.[98-103] Hypercapnia during anoxia in immature rats decreased consumption of high-energy phosphates.[104] Brain acidosis also inhibits NMDA receptor function, reduces glutamate levels, and decreases glutamate release, all of which can reduce excitatory amino acid neurotoxicity.[103,105-107] Extracellular acidosis decreases Ca^{2+} flux into the cell through both voltage-operated and receptor-operated Ca^{2+} channels, including that occurring in response to NMDA receptor activation.[107,108]

Calcium

Calcium is a crucial intracellular second messenger. It modulates the activity of numerous pathways and enzymes, including lipases, proteases, endonucleases, protein kinases, protein phosphatases, and mitochondrial dehydrogenases. As such, it also affects gene expression, protein synthesis, and cellular secretion. Intracellular Ca^{2+} concentration (Ca_i) is, therefore, controlled within a very narrow range under physiological circumstances.[109] Influx is regulated by voltage-operated and receptor-operated Ca^{2+} channels (i.e., the N-methyl-D-aspartate (NMDA) receptor). Intracellular sites of sequestration and release include endoplasmic reticulum and mitochondria. Calcium extrusion is accomplished by Ca-ATPases and a Na^+/Ca^{2+} exchanger, which is driven by the Na^+ gradient. Calcium influx across brain cell membranes can occur by activation of ionotropic glutamate receptors such as the NMDA receptor. Metatropic glutamate receptors, as well as those of numerous other agonists, are coupled to phospholipase C (PLC) and generate inositol triphosphate (IP_3), which provokes Ca^{2+}

release from intracellular stores, such as endoplasmic reticulum. Calcium entry can itself cause intracellular calcium release, a phenomenon known as calcium-triggered calcium release.[109] Under normal circumstances, increases in Ca_i are rapidly modulated by membrane extrusion and/or sequestration into endoplasmic reticulum, processes requiring ATP, and into mitochondria, which uses energy derived from the mitochondrial proton motive force.

Increases in Ca_i occur during hypoxia and ischemia. Multiple mechanisms are involved. These include acidosis-triggered release from endoplasmic reticulum and mitochondria, NMDA receptor-stimulated opening of receptor-operated Ca^{2+} channels by glutamate, opening of voltage-operated channels due to membrane depolarization, enhanced Na^+/Ca^{2+} exchange, and loss of ATP- and energy-dependent sequestration of calcium in mitochondria and of Ca/ATPase membrane pump activity. Increased free radical generation may compound these effects. Furthermore, many cytokines produced during bypass such as interleukin-8 and tumor necrosis factor-α,[110] can signal through receptors coupled to PLC, which will increase Ca_i by stimulating production of IP_3.[80] Increased calcium has been demonstrated in both immature and adult brain in response to hypoxia-ischemia, energetic depletion, and excitatory neurotransmitter stimulation.[80,111–113]

The consequences of calcium overload are multiple. They include *excessive* lipolysis, proteolysis, DNA fragmentation, further energetic depletion, and microtubular disassembly. Abnormal activation of protein kinase phosphorylation and/or phosphatases can alter gene expression, ion channel activity, perturb intracellular signaling pathways, and inhibit protein synthesis.[114–118] Altered gene expression may change protein synthesis and activate an apoptotic program. Calcium stimulates both oxyradical and nitric oxide-producing enzymes, thereby increasing free radical injury. Membrane damage from free radical-mediated lipid peroxidation and protein oxidation may promote receptor and ion channel dysfunction, thereby allowing further calcium entry.[114,119]

Excitatory Amino Acids

Excitatory and inhibitory amino acids are the most abundant neurotransmitters in the brain.[70,120] Glutamate (excitatory) and GABA inhibitory effect approximately 75% of brain transmissions. It is likely that all neurons can be stimulated by glutamate. Glutamate is the most abundant amino acid in the central nervous system, although only a small fraction is involved in neural transmission. However, this leaves a large pool, normally involved in intermediary metabolism, available for release during brain injury.[70]

Classification of excitatory amino acid (EAA) subtypes has been based upon receptor preference for synthetic agonists: NMDA, quisqualate, kainate, and α-amino-3-hydroxy-5-methyl-4-isoxazole (AMPA). There is now abundant evidence that EAA receptors are critical to numerous physiological processes in developing brain. These include regulation of neuronal growth and regression, axonal and dendritic development, and synapse formation.[70] In fact, transient overproduction of EAA synapses appears to be frequent during infancy, occurring in regions undergoing aggressive development, organization, synaptic stabilization, and synaptic elimination. This has been demonstrated in areas such as cerebral cortex, visual cortex, globus pallidus, and basal ganglia. In addition to neurotrophic functions, EAAs participate in the development of neuronal cytoarchitecture and circuitry. Another important feature may be regulation of synaptic plasticity, including forms of learning and memory related to long-term potentiation and experience-dependent plasticity. Blocking NMDA receptors appear to lead to decreased plasticity in experimental models.

As alluded to above, glutamate receptors not only serve trophic and maturational functions but also mediate the selective synaptic reduction that occurs in developing brain. This function may be at least as important as growth stimulation. Overall synaptic reduction will reduce "neuronal noise." It is also critical that the correct synapses be retained or eliminated.

It is thus clear that excessive activation of these same EAA pathways during various forms of cerebral injury such as hypoxia, ischemia, and trauma can produce neurotoxicity. Metabolic stress appears to be a major predisposing feature. In the initial phase of hypoxia or ischemia, ATP depletion causes reversed operation of membrane glutamate uptake carriers (i.e., glutamate is released), leading to increased and sustained activation of NMDA and AMPA receptors by glutamate. This results in membrane depolarization; influx of Na^+, Cl^-, and H_2O; and cell swelling. Intracellular Ca_i also increases due to glutamate-stimulated NMDA activity, resulting in sustained potentiation of NMDA receptor-gated currents, as well as activating numerous Ca-dependent processes (see above). Additional glutamate can be released during and after ischemia due to calcium-dependent exocytosis of glutamate; this triggers further NMDA-dependent calcium uptake and cellular injury.[111,112,121]

Neuronal injury can occur due to stimulation of the quisqualate metabotropic receptor. This receptor is linked to membrane phospholipase C, which breaks down membrane phospholipids to yield IP_3 and diacylglycerol (DAG). IP_3 promotes further calcium release from intracellular stores, whereas DAG activates the pluripotential protein kinase C (PKC). In addition to furthering calcium-mediated injury, membrane damage may occur from excessive stimulation of membrane phospholipases.[122] The role of PKC in brain injury remains controversial, with evidence suggesting that PKC is both protective[123,124] and harmful.[125]

Antagonists of EAA receptors can significantly reduce excitatory neurotoxicity in both adult and infant brain.[70,111,112,126-128] Efficacy has been shown when these antagonists are given before injury, as well as during the early recovery phase. Efficacy during the recovery phase may relate to preventing receptor stimulation caused by the exocytosis of additional glutamate described above. In infants, the potency of glutamate receptor subtypes to produce neurotoxicity is NMDA $\gg$ quisqualate/AMPA $>$ kainate, as compared to kainate $\gg$ NMDA $=$ quisqualate/AMPA in adults. It is thus likely that NMDA and/or NMDA plus AMPA inhibition would be most effective in infants, whereas an alternate strategy is required in mature brain. Differences in antagonist efficacy between focal and global ischemia models have also been observed.

Despite the experimental benefits seen in some models treated with NMDA or AMPA antagonists, as well as the close correlation often seen between EAA receptor density and brain injury, the protection afforded by these agents is often incomplete. Furthermore, not all regions with high EAA density are certain to be injured by hypoxia-ischemia or other insults and, conversely, areas with lower density can be vulnerable. It is thus likely that EAA density is one important factor in a matrix that involves local environment, blood flow, energy status, and other defense mechanisms against calcium overload and free radical injury.

Nonetheless, the pivotal role of EAA activity in normal brain development makes it a crucial consideration in the production of both acute and chronic neurological dysfunction after cardiopulmonary bypass and DHCA. A critical level of EAA stimulation is required for normal brain development in specific regions at specific times. Excessive activation may lead to generalized glutamate-induced excitotoxicity, as well as to altered neuronal development, integration, and plasticity. Too little activity may also compromise development. Thus, although it has been said that the increased plasticity of neonatal brain may operate in favor of the cardiac surgeon,[129] it appears at least as likely that mechanisms underlying the tremendous growth and remodeling potential of the immature brain may predispose it to neurological injury.

Free Radical Injury

If ATP depletion and its consequences are responsible for much of the sequelae of hypoxic-ischemic brain injury, free radical production is responsible for a significant portion of that occurring during reperfusion.[130-132] Reactive oxygen species, such as $\cdot O_2^-$ (superoxide), are intermediate or are byproducts of numerous oxidation reactions, particularly within mitochondria. In the presence of NADH (H^+) and the enzyme superoxide dismutase, hydrogen peroxide (H_2O_2) is formed from $\cdot O_2^-$. Hydrogen peroxide can be scavenged by catalase ($2H_2O_2 \rightarrow O_2 + 2H_2O$) and glutathione peroxidase (2 GSH + $H_2O_2 \rightarrow$ GSSG + $2H_2O_2$). However, in the presence of iron, production of the highly toxic and reactive hydroxyl ($\cdot OH^-$) species can occur:

$$\cdot O_2^- + Fe^{+3} \rightarrow Fe^{+2} + O_2^-$$
$$\underline{Fe^{+2} + H_2O_2 \rightarrow Fe^{+3} + OH^- + \cdot OH^- \quad \text{(fast)}}$$
$$\text{net:} \quad \cdot O_2^- + H_2O_2 \rightarrow O_2 + OH^- + \cdot OH^-$$

Under aerobic conditions, the "physiological" amounts of $\cdot OH^-$ produced are efficiently scavenged by endogenous substances, such as glutathione, vitamins C and E, and superoxide dismutase-catalase. Additionally, intracellular iron and calcium levels are under precise control, and NADH (H^+) is relatively low due to oxidative phosphorylation. Ischemia poises the cell for a burst of free radical production when O_2 is resupplied, because intracellular H^+, free iron, and calcium concentration all increase during ischemia. Glutathione and other antioxidants are often depleted very early during reperfusion. Furthermore, prematurity, nutritional deficiency, and cyanosis may be associated with diminished antioxidant reserves.[133-138]

Additional $\cdot O_2^-$ can be generated by the actin of cyclooxygenase and lipoxygenase during the formation of prostaglandins and leukotrienes, respectively, from arachidonic acid arising from the breakdown of membrane phospholipids. Purine catabolites, such as hypoxanthine, accumulate in ischemic tissue due to ATP hydrolysis and nucleic acid catabolism. Under aerobic conditions, hypoxanthine and xanthine are converted to uric acid and NADH (H^+) by xanthine dehydrogenase. During ischemia, a calcium-activated protease converts xanthine dehydrogenase to xanthine oxidase, such that hypoxanthine and xanthine are converted to $\cdot O_2^-$ plus uric acid.[80]

The oxyradicals thus formed attack membrane lipids and proteins, injuring both vascular endothelium and parenchymal cells. Free radicals also inhibit EAA uptake, as well as enhance release, thereby exacerbating neurotoxicity.[114] The resultant membrane dysfunction can set up a cycle of reduced perfusion (due to vascular injury), edema, lipid peroxidation, calcium overload, and further oxyradical formation and cell injury.[139–142]

Despite significant evidence supporting the central role of free radicals in reperfusion injury, efforts to reduce their production have met with mixed success in terms of changing outcome. Inhibition of xanthine oxidase (e.g., allopurinol), $\cdot O_2^-$ scavenging (exogenous superoxide dismutase with or without catalase), administration of intracellular superoxide dismutase mimics (e.g., tempol), iron chelation (deferoxamine), and lazaroids (21-aminosteroids) have all had variable efficacy.[143–147] In general, antioxidant strategies have been more effective when administered before and/or during ischemia-reperfusion, which may have some relevance to planned circulatory arrest.

Nitric Oxide

Constitutive isoforms of NO exist in brain endothelial cells and certain neurons. In endothelium, NO· regulates vascular tone and perfusion by its ability to stimulate smooth muscle guanylate cyclase to produce cyclic guanosine monophosphate (cGMP), promoting relaxation. NO· also decreases white cell and platelet adhesion to endothelium. Endothelial cells release NO· under basal conditions and in response to factors such as shear stress, adenosine diphosphate (ADP), thrombin, endothelin, acetylcholine, bradykinin, and serotonin. Calcium is a required cofactor, and increased endothelial Ca_i is thought to be a common messenger stimulating endothelial NO· synthase, which catalyzes the formation of from NO· from L-arginine and O_2.[148]

A structurally distinct, constitutively present NO· synthase enzyme is located in multiple (but not all) neuronal cell populations and is believed to act as a neurotransmitter and modulate neuronal development and plasticity. Interestingly, some aspects of memory and behavior may also be served by brain *endothelial* NO· synthase.[149,150] The neuronal enzyme is also activated by calcium. Numerous studies have linked EAA-stimulated NMDA activation, increased Ca_i, NO· production, and the development of brain injury.[112,148,151,152] A third NO· synthase isoform is induced over several hours by cytokines such as interferon-g and tumor necrosis factor-α in brain macrophages and microglial cells; this isoform is not constitutively present, is not regulated by calcium, and produces significantly larger amounts of NO·. Proinflammatory cytokines also induce the synthesis of other potential neurotoxins, such as quinolinic acid.[153]

Possible mechanisms of NO^--mediated neuronal toxicity are multiple NO· binds avidly to iron-containing proteins. Important consequences include inhibition of enzymes such as aconitase (Krebs cycle), iron-sulfur centers mediating mitochondrial transport, and ribonucleotide reductase. It is likely that NO·, either directly or indirectly, affects many types of gene expression, protein synthesis, and receptor function. NO· can also react with superoxide to form the peroxynitrite radical (·ONOO⁻), which may be toxic itself and form ·OH⁻ in the presence of H^+.[96] However, ·ONOO⁻ can also rearrange to yield nontoxic NO_2^-, and thus NO^- scavenging of ·O_2^- might be protective under certain conditions.

Experimentally, both protective and injurious effects from NO in the brain have been demonstrated. Protective effects from NO, likely to be of endothelial origin, have been linked to maintenance of cerebral blood flow and inhibition of white cell and platelet function. On the other hand, EAA-stimulated NO synthesis and deleterious interaction with superoxide have also been shown, as has neuronal toxicity from cytokine-stimulated NO production in the brain.[151,153–157]

INFLAMMATORY CELLS AND MEDIATORS

Cardiopulmonary bypass causes a systemic inflammatory response due to several factors, which include surgical trauma, blood contact with the CPB circuit, and ischemia-reperfusion injury.[158–162] These events stimulate a complex and often interconnected series of events that include activation of the coagulation, fibrinolytic, and complement pathways; endotoxin release and cytokine production; oxygen and nitric oxide radical production; expression of leukocyte adhesion molecules on the endothelial surface; and activation of neutrophils, with release of free radicals and proteolytic enzymes.

Activation of the contact limb of the coagulation cascade (and particularly factor XIIa) leads to neutrophil activation, degranulation, and elastase release.[163,164] Fibrin degradation products arising from fibrinolytic activity impair platelet function and disrupt endothelial cells.

Production of complement fragments during bypass can occur due to stimulation of the alternate pathway by foreign surface contact, endotoxin, and kallikrein. Protamine can activate the classical pathway. Indices of complement activity increase three- to five-fold with initiation of bypass, and they increase 2 to 3 times higher still during the rewarming and reperfusion phase.[159] Blood concentrations of C3a and perhaps C5b correlate with postbypass renal, cardiac, and pulmonary dysfunction.[158] Various complement fragments induce smooth muscle constriction, platelet activation and aggregation, histamine release, white cell activation, free radical production and degranulation, and capillary leak. Terminal complement fragments can incorporate into the cell membrane and direct cell lysis.

Neutrophil activation is a recurrent theme of the inflammatory response to cardiopulmonary bypass. It is produced by a wide variety of stimuli, including foreign surface contact, endotoxin, complement, cytokines, platelet-activating factor (PAF), and ischemia-reperfusion. Activated neutrophils express proadhesive molecules on their cell surface, migrate into tissue, have increased lipoxygenase and myeloperoxidase activity (sources of $\cdot O_2^-$ and hypochlorous acid, respectively), and release elastase and other proteolytic enzymes. These events damage membrane lipids, proteins, and DNA. Elastase can also cause endothelial injury, inactivate serine proteases in the coagulation pathways, and cleave the proadhesive Gp-Ib receptor off of the platelet membrane.[164,165]

Blood bacterial endotoxin concentrations can be increased during bypass, perhaps by reduced intestinal perfusion. Endotoxin can directly injure endothelial cells, causing capillary leak, as well as stimulate the production of proinflammatory cytokines, such as tumor necrosis factor-α (TNF-α), interleukin-1β (IL-1β), IL-6, and IL-8. Circulating levels of one or more of these substances are increased during CPB.[110,158,163] Cytokine production can also be stimulated by foreign surface contact, complement fragments, and other cytokines. Mechanisms of cytokine-induced tissue injury are multiple.

Cytokines such as IL-1β and TNF-α are directly toxic to endothelial and other cells via mechanisms that may include NO· production, apoptosis, and enhanced free radical injury. Cytokine-induced vascular smooth muscle NO· production can result in profound hypotension (e.g., septic shock).[148] IL-1β and TNF-α cause wasting and edema. Local production of IL-8 occurs as a consequence of ischemia-reperfusion and stimulation by other cytokines. IL-8 promotes leukocytosis, neutrophil chemotaxis, and activation of neutrophil proteases and free radical enzymes. Modified hemofiltration reduces concentrations of some complement fragments and those of IL-6 and TNF-α; improvements in blood loss, time to extubation, hemodynamics, and cerebral metabolic recovery have been associated with ultrafiltration.[110,166]

TNF-α (alone or in potentiated fashion with other cytokines, such as IL-1 or interferon-γ) can induce brain nitric oxide synthesis, as well as stimulate expression of leukocyte adhesion molecules on the endothelial surface.[167] NO· production may be toxic to the brain by free radical interaction and inhibition of oxidative metabolism, as described previously. Leukocyte activation, adhesion, and migration into the brain may allow further neutrophil-mediated injury. TNF-α stimulates glial cells and thus regulates gliosis, tissue remodeling, and scar formation.[167] Finally, cytokines may alter cell function and gene expression by means of other mechanisms that stimulate second messenger pathways, such as phospholipase C, protein kinase C, tyrosine kinases, and protein phosphatases.[168] TNF-α also induces apoptosis in certain cell types, in part by means of a mechanism involving mitochondrial free radical production.[169]

The cellular limb of the immune system may participate in mediating brain injury under conditions relevant to bypass. The Fas antigen is a member of a cell surface protein superfamily that includes the NGF receptor, TNF receptor, and certain T- and B-cell antigens.[170] Stimulation of Fas receptor by Fas ligand, typically present in T cells, can trigger apoptosis in Fas antigen-positive cells.[171] One physiological role of the Fas antigen-antibody system is the deletion of autoreactive T cells.[172] However, hypoxia and, perhaps, cytokines induce Fas antigen expression on nonimmune cells.[173] The importance of this mechanism of apoptotic cell death in reperfused and inflamed brain remains to be seen.

OTHER CONSIDERATIONS

As noted above, the genetic program is important to brain development. Molecular biology techniques are beginning to elucidate genetic bases of CHD. For example, the association of conotruncal defects, DiGeorge and velocardiofacial syndrome, and microdeletion of chromosome 22 has been reported.[174] Many, if not all, of these patients have some degree of developmental delay. Thus, "postoperative" neurological dysfunction may be genetically predetermined in some of our patients.

The numerous beneficial effects of hypothermia are several and well-accepted. Of particular relevance to the present discussion, hypothermia reduces leukocyte-endothelial interaction and decreases inflammatory cell injury.[175] The literature on the protective effects of hypothermia against brain ischemia is substantial. Nonetheless, even this standard therapy may warrant further examination as a *cause* of delayed brain injury, particularly in the developing brain, as hypothermia at nonfreezing temperatures can induce apoptosis in cultured cells.[176]

References

1. Jenkins KJ, Newburger JW, Lock JE, Davis RB, Coffman GA, Iezzoni LI: In-hospital mortality for surgical repair of congenital heart defects: Preliminary observations of variation by hospital caseload. Pediatrics 95: 323–330, 1995
2. Berthrong M, Sabiston DC: Cerebral lesions in congenital heart disease: a review of autopsies on one hundred and sixty-two cases. Bull Johns Hopkins Hosp 89:384–401, 1951

3. Glauser TA, Rorke LB, Weinberg PM, Clancy RR: Congenital brain anomalies associated with the hypoplastic left heart syndrome. Pediatrics 85: 984–990, 1990
4. Terplan KL: Patterns of brain damage in infants and children with congenital heart disease. Am J Dis Child 125:175, 1973
5. Ferry PC: Neurological sequelae of open-heart surgery in children: An "irritating question." Am J Dis Child 44:369–373, 1990
6. Glauser TA, Rorke LB, Weinberg PM, Clancy RR: Acquired neuropathologic lesions associated with the hypoplastic left heart syndrome. Pediatrics 85:991–1000, 1990
6a. Villano ME, O'Brien JJ, Morris KJ: Embolic events recorded during pediatric cardiopulmonary bypass. Presented at The 3rd International Conference, The Brain and Cardiac Surgery, Key West, Florida, September 24, 1994
7. Newburger JW, Jonas RA, Wernovsky G: A comparison of the perioperative neurologic effects of hypothermic circulatory arrest versus low-flow cardiopulmonary bypass in infant heart surgery. N Engl J Med 329: 1057–1064, 1993
8. Greeley WJ, Ungerleider RM, Kern FH, Brusino FG, Smith LR, Reves JG: Effects of cardiopulmonary bypass on cerebral blood flow in neonates, infants, and children. Circulation 80 (suppl I):209–215, 1989
9. Greeley WJ, Kern FH, Ungerleider RM et al: The effect of hypothermic cardiopulmonary bypass and total circulatory arrest on cerebral metabolism in neonates, infants, and children. J Thorac Cardiovasc Surg 101: 783–794, 1991
10. Greeley WJ, Bracey VA, Ungerleider RM et al: Recovery of cerebral metabolism and mitochondrial oxidation state is delayed after hypothermic circulatory arrest. Circulation 84 (suppl III):400–406, 1991
11. Greeley WJ, Ungerleider RM: Assessing the effect of cardiopulmonary bypass on the brain. Ann Thorac Surg 52:417–419, 1991
12. Newburger JW, Silbert AR, Buckley LP, Flyer DC: Cognitive function and age at repair of transposition of the great arteries in children. N Engl J Med 310:1495–1499, 1984
13. Schell RM, Kern FH, Greeley WG et al: Cerebral blood flow and metabolism during cardiopulmonary bypass. Anesth Analg 76:849–865, 1993
14. Swain JA, Anderson RV, Siegman MG: Low flow cardiopulmonary bypass and brain protection: A summary of investigations. Ann Thorac Surg, in press, 1996
15. Griepp EB, Griepp RB: Cerebral consequences of hypothermic circulatory arrest in adult. J Cardiac Surg 7:134–155, 1992
16. Michenfelder JD: The hypothermic brain. In Anesthesia and the Brain, pp. 23–24. New York, Churchill Livingstone, 1988
17. Kern FH, Jonas RA, Mayer JE Jr, Hanley FL, Castaneda AR, Hickey PR: Temperature monitoring during CPB in infants: Does it predict efficient brain cooling? Ann Thorac Surg 54:749–754, 1992
18. Foster JMT, Burrows FA, Bissonnette B: Brain temperature during low flow hypothermic cardiopulmonary bypass. Anesthesiology 79:A1144, 1993
19. Kern FH, Ungerleider RM, Schulman S et al: Comparison of two strategies of CPB cooling on jugular venous oxygen saturation. Anesthesiology 33:A1136, 1992
20. Mault JR, Ohtake S, Klingensmith M, Heinle JS, Greeley WJ, Ungerleider RM: Cerebral metabolism and circulatory arrest: Effects of duration and strategies for protection. Ann Thorac Surg 55:57–64, 1993

21. Bellinger DC, Wernovsky G, Rappaport LA et al: Cognitive development of children following early repair of transposition of the great arteries using deep hypothermic circulatory arrest. Pediatrics 87:701–707, 1991
22. Becker H, Vinten-Johansen J, Buckberg GD et al: Myocardial damage caused by keeping pH 7.40 during systemic deep hypothermia. J Thoracic Cardiovasc Surg 82:810–820, 1981
23. Bove EL, West HL, Paskanik AM: Hypothermic cardiopulmonary bypass: A comparison between alpha stat and pH stat regulation in the dog. J Surg Res 42:66–73, 1987
24. Kern FH, Ungerleider RM, Quill TJ et al: Cerebral blood flow response to changes in arterial carbon dioxide during hypothermic cardiopulmonary bypass in children. J Thorac Cardiovasc Surg 101:618–622, 1991
25. Murkin JM, Farrar JK, Tweed WA, McKenzie FN, Guiraudon G: Cerebral autoregulation and flow/metabolism coupling during cardiopulmonary bypass: The influence of $Paco_2$. Anesth Analg 66:825–832, 1987
26. Nevin M, Colchester AC, Adams S, Pepper JR: Evidence for involvement of hypocapnia and hypoperfusion in aetiology of neurological deficit after cardiopulmonary bypass. Lancet 2:1493–1495, 1987
27. Nevin M, Pepper JR: Carbon dioxide, brain damage, and cardiac surgery [Letter]. Lancet 1:949, 1988
28. Prough DS, Stump DA, Roy RC et al: Response of cerebral blood flow to changes in carbon dioxide tension during hypothermic cardiopulmonary bypass. Anesthesiology 64:576–581, 1986
29. Jonas RA, Bellinger DC, Rappaport LA et al: Relation of pH strategy and developmental outcome after hypothermic circulatory arrest. J Thorac Cardiovasc Surg 106:362–368, 1993
30. Bayley N: Manual for the Bayley Scales of Infant Development, 2nd ed. San Antonio, TX, Psychological Corporation, 1993
31. McCarthy D: McCarthy Scales of Children's Abilities. New York, The Psychological Corporation, 1972
32. Shewmon DA: What is a neonatal seizure? Problems in definition and quantification for investigative and clinical purposes. J Clin Neurophysiol 7:315–368, 1993
33. Volpe JJ: Neonatal seizures: Current concepts and revised classification. Pediatrics 84:422–428, 1989
34. Scher MS, J PM: Controversies concerning neonatal seizures. Pediatr Clin North Am 36:281–310, 1989
35. Zelnik N, Nir A, Amit S, Iancu TC: Autonomic seizures in an infant: Unusual cutaneous and cardiac manifestations. Dev Med Child Neurol 32:74–78, 1990
36. Clancy RR, Legido A, Lewis D: Occult neonatal seizures. Epilepsia 29:256–261, 1988
37. Ehyai A, Fenichel GM, Bender HW Jr: Incidence and prognosis of seizures in infants after cardiac surgery with profound hypothermia and circulatory arrest. JAMA 252:3165–3167, 1984
38. Wical BS, Tomasi LG: A distinctive neurologic syndrome after induced profound hypothermia. Pediatr Neurol 6:202–205, 1990
39. DeLeon S, Ilbawa M, Arcilla R et al: Choreoathetosis after deep hypothermia without circulatory arrest. Ann Thorac Surg 50:714–719, 1990
40. Brunberg JA, Reilly D, Doty DB: Choreoathetosis in infants following cardiac surgery with deep hypothermia and circulatory arrest. J Pediatr 84:232–235, 1974

41. Almond CH, Jones JC, Snyder HM et al: Cooling gradients and brain damage with deep hypothermia. J Thorac Cardiovasc Surg 48:890–897, 1964
42. Norwood WI, Norwood CR, Castaneda AR: Cerebral anoxia: Effect of deep hypothermia and pH. Surgery 86:203–209, 1979
43. Ames AI, Wright RL, Kowada M, Thurston AB, Majno G: Cerebral ischemia the no reflow phenomenon. Am J Pathol 52:437–447, 1968
44. Robinson RO, Samuels M, Pohl KRE: Choreic syndrome after cardiac surgery. Arch Dis Child 63:1466–1469, 1988
45. Wong PC, Barlow CF, Hickey PR et al: Factors associated with choreoathetosis after cardiopulmonary bypass in children with congenital heart disease. Circulation 86 (suppl II):118–126, 1992
46. Blackwood MJA, Haka-Ikse K, Steward DJ: Developmental outcome in children undergoing surgery with profound hypothermia. Anesthesiology 65:437–440, 1986
47. Clarkson PM, MacArthur BA, Barratt-Boyes BG, Whitlock RM, Neutze JM: Developmental progress after cardiac surgery in infancy using hypothermia and circulatory arrest. Circulation 62:855–861, 1980
48. Wells FC, Coghill S, Caplan HL, Lincoln C: Duration of circulatory arrest does influence the psychological development of children after cardiac operations in early life. J Thorac Cardiovasc Surg 86:823–831, 1983
49. Wright JS, Hicks RG, Newman DC: Deep hypothermic arrest: Observations on later development in children. J Thorac Cardiovasc Surg 77: 466–468, 1979
50. Haka-Ikse K, Blackwood M, Steward DJ: Psychomotor development of infants and children after profound hypothermia during surgery for congenital heart disease. Dev Med Child Neurol 20:62–70, 1978
51. Bellinger DC, Jonas RA, Rappaport LA et al: Developmental and neurologic status of children after heart surgery with hypothermic circulatory arrest or low-flow cardiopulmonary bypass. N Engl J Med 332: 549–555, 1995
52. Lanier WL, Stangland KJ, Scheithauer BW, Milde JH, Michenfelder JD: The effects of dextrose infusion and head position on neurologic outcome after complete cerebral ischemia in primates: Examination of a model. Anesthesiology 66:33–48, 1987
53. Lanzino G, Kassell NF, Germanson T, Truskowski L, Alves W: Plasma glucose levels and outcome after aneurysmal subarachnoid hemorrhage. J Neurosurg 79:885–891, 1993
54. Nakakimura K, Fleischer JE, Drummond JC et al: Glucose administration before cardiac arrest worsens neurologic outcome in cats. Anesthesiology 72:1005–1011, 1990
55. Pulsinelli W, Levy DE, Sigbee B et al: Increased damage after ischemic stroke in patients with hyperglycemia with or without established diabetes mellitus. Am J Med 74:540–544, 1983
56. Lanier WL: Glucose management during cardiopulmonary bypass: Cardiovascular and neurologic implications. Anesth Analg 72:423–427, 1991
57. Sieber FE, Smith DA, Traystman RJ, Wollman H: Glucose: A reevaluation of its intraoperative use. Anesthesiology 67:72–81, 1987
58. Steward DJ, DaSilva CA, Flegel T: Elevated blood glucose levels may increase the danger of neurological deficit following profoundly hypothermic cardiac arrest [Letter]. Anesthesiology 68:653, 1988

59. Hickey PR, Jonas RA, Wernovsky G et al: Blood glucose and perioperative neurologic outcome in infants undergoing cardiac surgery with hypothermic circulatory arrest. Anesthesiology, in press, 1996
60. Laptook AR, Corbett RJ, Nunnally RL: Effect of plasma glucose concentration on cerebral metabolism during partial ischemia in neonatal piglets. Stroke 21:435–440, 1990
61. Vannucci RC, Mujsce DJ: Effect of glucose on perinatal hypoxic-ischemic brain damage. Biol Neonate 62:215–224, 1992
62. Voorhies TM, Rawlinson D, Vannucci RC: Glucose and perinatal hypoxic-ischemic brain damage in the rat. Neurology 36:1115–1118, 1986
63. de Courten-Myers GM, Kleinholz M, Wagner KR, Myers RE: Normoglycemia (not hypoglycemia) optimizes outcome from middle cerebral artery occlusion. J Cereb Blood Flow Metab 14:227–236, 1994
64. Callahan DJ, Engle MJ, Volpe JJ: Hypoxic injury to developing glial cells: Protective effect of high glucose. Pediatr Res 27:186–190, 1990
65. Hattori H, Wasterlain CG: Post-hypoxic glucose supplement reduces hypoxic-ischemic damage in the neonatal rat. Ann Neurol 28:122–128, 1990
66. Lou HC: Hypoxic-hemodynamic pathogenesis of brain lesions in the newborn. Brain Dev 16:423–431, 1994
67. Affi AK, Bergman RA: Basic Neuroscience. Baltimore, Urban & Schwartzberg, 1986
68. Cowan WM: Aspects of neural development. In Porter R (ed): Neurophysiology III. International Review of Physiology, vol. 17, pp. 149–191. Baltimore, University Park Press
69. Bayer SA, Altman J: Neocortical Development. New York, Raven Press, 1991
70. McDonald JW, Johnston MV: Physiological and pathophysiological roles of excitatory amino acids during central nervous system development. Brain Res Rev 15:41–70, 1990
71. Steward O: Principles of Cellular, Molecular and Developmental Neuroscience. New York, Springer-Verlag, 1989
72. Hamburger V: Cell death in the development of the lateral motor column of the chick embryo. J Comp Neurol 160:535, 1975
73. Levi-Montalcini R, Levi G: Selective growth-stimulating effects of mouse sarcoma, producing hyperplasia of sympathetic ganglia and hyperneurotization of viscera in the chick embryo. J Exp Zool 123:223, 1953
74. Lee S, Christakos S, Small MB: Apoptosis and signal transduction: Clues to a molecular mechanism. Curr Opinion Cell Biol 5:286–291, 1993
75. Hopkin K: Programmed cell death: A switch to the cytoplasm? J Natl Inst Res 7:39–41, 1995
76. Horvitz HR, Ellis HM, Sternberg PW: Programmed cell death in nematode development. Neurosci Comment 1:56, 1982
77. Yuan JY, Horvitz HR: The Caenorhabditis elegans geens CED-3 and CED-4 act cell autonomously to cause programmed cell death. Dev Biol 138: 33, 1990
78. Linnik MD, Zobrist RH, Hatfield MD: Evidence supporting a role for programmed cell death in focal cerebral ischemia in rats. Stroke 24: 2002–2009, 1993
79. Gottlieb RA, Burleson KO, Koner RA: Reperfusion injury indices apoptosis in rabbit cardiomyotes. JCI 94:1621–1628, 1994
80. Vannucci RC: Experimental biology of cerebral hypoxia-ischemia: Relation to perinatal brain damage. Pediatr Res 27:317–326, 1990

81. Kawata, H, Fackler JC, Aoki M: Recovery of cerebral blood flow and energy state in piglets after hypothermic circulatory arrest versus recovery after low-flow bypass. J Thorac Cardiovasc Surg 106:671–685, 1993

82. Linn F, Paschen W, Grosse Ophoff B, Hossman K-A: Mitochondrial respiration during recirculation after prolonged ischemia in cat brain. Exp Neurol 96:321–333, 1987

83. Corbett RJT: In vivo multicenter magnetic resonance spectroscopy investigation of cerebral development. Semin Perinatol 14:258–262, 1990

84. Holtzman D, Olson J, Zamvil S: Maturation of potassium-stimulated respiration in rat cerebral cortex slices. J Neurochem 39:274–279, 1982

85. Holtzman D, McFarland EW, Jacobs D et al: Maturational increase in mouse brain creatine kinase rates shown by phosphorus magnetic resonance. Dev Brain Res 22:58–65, 1991

86. Kalimo H, Rehncrona S, Soderfeldt B, Olsson Y, Siesjo BK: Brain lactic acidosis and ischemic cell damage. II. Histopathology. J Cereb Blood Flow Metab 1:297–311, 1981

87. LeBlanc MH, Huang M, Patel D, Smith EE, Davidas M: Glucose given after hypoxic ischemia does not affect brain injury in piglets. Stroke 25:1443–1447, 1994

88. Michaud LJ, Rivara FP, Longstreth WT Jr, Grady MS: Elevated initial blood glucose levels and poor outcome following severe brain injuries in children. Trauma 31:1356–1362, 1991

89. Gardiner M, Smith M, Kagstrom E: Influence of blood glucose concentration on brain lactate accumulation during severe hypoxia and subsequent recovery of brain energy metabolism. J Cereb Blood Flow Metab 2:429–438, 1982

90. Moore TJ, Lione AP, Regen DM, Tarpley HL, Raines PL: Brain glucose metabolism in the newborn rat. Am J Physiol 221:1746–1753, 1971

91. Vannucci RC, Vasta F, Vannucci SJ: Cerebral metabolic responses of hyperglycemia immature rats to hypoxia-ischemia. Pediatr Res 21:524–529, 1987

92. Vannucci RC, Christensen MA, Stein DT: Regional cerebral glucose utilization in the immature rat: Effect of hypoxia-ischemia. Pediatr Res 26:208–214, 1989

93. Welsh FA: Regional evaluation of ischemic metabolic alterations. J Cereb Blood Flow Metab 4:309–316, 1984

94. Barry MA, Eastman A: Identification of deoxyribonuclease II as an endonuclease involved in apoptosis. Arch Biochem Biophys 300:440–450, 1993

95. Siesjo BK, Bendek G, Koide T et al: Influence of acidosis in lipid peroxidation in brain tissues in vitro. J Cereb Blood Flow Metabol 5:253–258, 1985

96. Beckman J, Meckman T, Chen J et al: Apparent hydroxyl radical production by peroxynitrite: Implications for endothelial injury from nitric oxide and superoxide. Proc Natl Acad Sci USA 87:1620–1624, 1990

97. Vannucci RC, Towfighi J, Heitjan DF, Brucklacher RB: Carbon dioxide protects the perinatal brain from hypoxic-ischemic damage: An experimental study in the immature rat. Pediatrics 95:868–874, 1995

98. Kogure K, Bjusto R, Scheinbert P, Reinmuth O: Dynamics of cerebral metabolism during moderate hypercapnia. J Neurochem 24:471–478, 1975

99. Miller AL, Corddry DH: Brain carbohydrate metabolism in developing rats during hypercapnia. J Neurochem 36:1202–1210, 1981
100. Miller AL, Hawkins RA, Veech RL: Decreased rate of glucose utilization by rat brain *in vivo* after exposure to atmospheres containing high concentrations of CO_2. J Neurochem 25:553–558, 1975
101. Berntman L, Dahlgren N, Siesjo BK: Cerebral blood flow and oxygen consumption in the rat brain during extreme hypercarbia. Anesthesiology 50:299–305, 1979
102. Folbergrova J, Ponten U, Siesjo BK: Patterns of changes in brain carbohydrate metabolites, amino acids and organic phosphates at increased carbon dioxide tensions. J Neurochem 22:1115–1125, 1974
103. Folbergrova J, Norberg K, Quistorff B, Siesjo BK: Carbohydrate and amino acid metabolism in rat cerebral cortex in moderate and extreme hypercapnia. J Neurochem 25:457–462, 1975
104. Vannucci RC, Duffy TE: Cerebral oxidative and energy metabolism of fetal and neonatal rats during anoxia and recovery. Am J Physiol 230: 1269–1275, 1976
105. Tombaugh GC, Sapolsky RM: Evolving concepts about the role of acidosis in ischemic neuropathology. J Neurochem 61:793–803, 1993
106. Kaku DA, Giffard RG, Choi DW: Neuroprotective effects of glutamate antagonists and extracellular acidity. Science 260:1516–1518, 1993
107. Takadera T, Shimada Y, Mohri T: Extracellular pH modulates N-methyl-D-aspartate receptor mediated neurotoxicity and calcium accumulation in rat cortical cultures. Brain Res 572:126–131, 1992
108. Ou-Yang Y, Kristian T, Mellergard P et al: The influence of pH on glutamate- and depolarization-induced increase of intracellular calcium concentration in cortical neurons in primary culture. Brain Res 646:65–72, 1994
109. Carafoli E: Intracellular calcium homeostasis. Annu Rev Biochem 56: 395–433, 1987
110. Journois D, Pouard P, Greeley WJ, Mauriat P et al: Hemofiltration during cardiopulmonary bypass in pediatric cardiac surgery. Effects on hemostasis, cytokines, and complement components. Anesthesiology 81: 1181–1189, 1996
111. Choi DW: Glutamate neurotoxicity and disease of the nervous system. Neuron 1:623–634, 1988
112. Choi DW: Calcium: Still center-stage in hypoxic-ischemic neuronal death. Trends Neurosci 18:58–60, 1995
113. Stein DT, Vannucci RC: Calcium accumulation during the evolution of hypoxic-ischemic brain damage in the immature rat. J Cereb Blood Flow Metabol 8:834–842, 1988
114. Siesjo BK, Katsura K-I, Kristian T: The biochemical basis of cerebral ischemic damage. J Neurosurg Anesth 7:47–52, 1995
115. Deshpande JK, Siesjo BK, Wieloch T: Calcium accumulation and neuronal damage in the rat hippocampus following cerebral ischemia. J Cereb Blood Flow Metab, 7:89–95, 1987
116. Widmann R, Weber C, Bonnekoh P, Schlenker M, Hossmann K-A: Neuronal damage after repeated 5 minutes ischemia in the gerbil is preceded by prolonged impairment of protein metabolism. J Cereb Blood Flow Metab 12:425–433, 1992
117. Umemura A, Mabe H, Nagai HA: Phospholipase-C inhibitor ameliorates postischemic neuronal damage in rats. Stroke 23:1163–1166, 1992

118. Wieloch T, Bergstedt K, Hu BR: Protein phosphorylation and the regulation of mRNA translation following cerebral ischemia. Prog Brain Res 96:179–191, 1993
119. Orrenius S, Burkitt MJ, Kass GEN et al: Calcium ions and oxidative cell injury. Ann Neurol 32:S33–S42, 1992
120. McDonald JW, Silverstein FS, Johnston MV: Neurotoxicity of N-methyl-D-aspartate is markedly enhanced in developing rat central nervous system. Brain Res 459:200–203, 1988
121. Szatkowski M, Attwell D: Triggering and execution of neuronal cell death in brain ischaemia: Two phases of glutamate release by different mechanisms. Trends Neurosci 17:359–365, 1994
122. Berridge MJ: Inositol triphosphate and diacylglycerol: Two interacting second messengers. Annu Rev Biochem 56:615, 1987
123. Zivin JA, Kochhar A, Saitoh T. Protein phosphorylation during ischemia. Stroke 21(suppl III):III117–III121, 1990
124. Madden KP, Clark WM, Kochhar A, Zivin JA: Effect of protein kinase C modulation on outcome of experimental CNS ischemia. Brain Res 547:193–198, 1991
125. Maiese K, Boniece IR, Skurat K, Wagner JA: Protein kinases modulate the sensitivity of hippocampal neurons to nitric oxide toxicity and anoxia. J Neurosci Res 36:77–87, 1993
126. McDonald JW, Silverstein FS, Johnston MV: MK-801 protects the neonatal brain from hypoxic-ischemic damage. Eur J Pharmacol 140:359–361, 1987
127. McDonald JW, Silverstein FS, Johnston MV: Neuroprotective effects of MK-801, TCP, PCP and CPP against N-methyl-D-aspartate induced neurotoxicity in an in vivo perinatal rat model. Brain Res 490:33–40, 1989
128. Pulsinelli W, Sarokin A, Buchan A: Antagonism of the NMDA and non-NMDA receptors in global versus focal brain ischemia. Prog Brain Res 96:125–135, 1993
129. Castaneda AR, Jonas RA, Mayer JE Jr, Hanley FL: Cardiac Surgery of the Neonate and Infant, p. 8. Philadelphia, WB Saunders, 1994
130. Bolli R: Mechanism of myocardial stunning. Circulation 82:723–738, 1990
131. Sakomoto A, Ohnishi ST, Ohnishi T, Ogawa R: Relationship between free-radical production and lipid peroxidation during ischemia-reperfusion injury in the rat brain. Brain Res 554:186–192, 1991
132. Traystman RJ, Kirsch JR, Koehler RC: Oxygen radical mechanism of brain injury following ischemia and reperfusion. J Appl Physiol 71:1185–1195, 1991
133. Cowan DB, Weisel RD, Williams WG, Mickle DA: The regulation of glutathione peroxidase gene expression by oxygen tension in cultured human cardiomyocytes. J Mol Cell Cardiol 24:423–433, 1992
134. Li R-K, Shaikh N, Wisel RD, Williams WG, Mickle DAG: Oxyradial-induced antioxidant and lipid changes in cultures human cardiomyocytes. Am J Physiol 266:H2204–H2211, 1994
135. Inder TE, Graham P, Sanderson K, Taylor BJ: Lipid peroxidation as a measure of oxygen free radical damage in the very low birthweight infant. Arch Dis Childh (Fetal Neonatal Edition) 70:F107–F111, 1994
136. Frank L, Sosenko IR: Development of lung antioxidant enzyme system in late gestation: Possible implications for the prematurely born infant. J Pediatr 110:9–14, 1987
137. Frank L: Antioxidants, nutrition, and bronchopulmonary dysplasia. Clin Perinatol 19:541–562, 1992

138. Litov RE, Coombs GF Jr: Selenium in pediatric nutrition. Pediatrics 87: 339–351, 1991
139. Chan PH, Schmidley JW, Fishman RA, Longar SM: Brain injury, edema and vascular permeability changes induced by oxygen-derived free radicals. Neurology 34:315–320, 1984
140. Rosenberg AA, Murdaugh E, White CW: The role of oxygen free radicals in post asphyxia cerebral hypoperfusion in newborn lambs. Pediatr Res 26:215–219, 1989
141. Patt A, Harken AH, Burton LM, Rodell TC et al: Xanthine oxidase-derived hydrogen peroxide contributes to ischemia reperfusion-induced edema in gerbil brains. J Clin Invest 81:1556–1562, 1988
142. Palmer C, Vannucci RC: Potential new therapies for perinatal cerebral hypoxia-ischemia. Clin Perinatol 20:411–432, 1993
143. Martz D, Rayos G, Schielke GP, Betz AL: Allopurinol and dimethylthiourea reduce brain infarction following middle cerebral artery occlusion in rats. Stroke 20:488–494, 1989
144. Hall ED, Pazara KE, Braughler MJ: 21-Aminosteroid lipid peroxidation inhibitor U74006F protects against cerebral ischemia in gerbils. Stroke 19: 997–1002, 1988
145. Mickle DA, Li R-K, Weisel RD, Birnbaum PL et al: Myocardial salvage with trolox and ascorbic acid for an acute evolving infarction. Ann Thorac Surg 47:553–557, 1989
146. Palmer C, Vannucci RC, Towfighi J, DuPlessis AJ, Vickers F: Allopurinol reduces hypoxic-ischemic brain injury. Pediatr Res 27:332–336, 1990
147. Hara H, Kogure K, Kato H, Ozaki A, Sukamoto T: Amelioration of brain damage after focal ischemia in the rat by a novel inhibitor of lipid peroxidation. Eur J Pharmacol 197:75–82, 1991
148. Moncada S, Palmer RMJ, Higgs EA: Nitric oxide: Physiology, pathophysiology, and pharmacology. Pharmacol Rev 43:109–138, 1991
149. Bredt DS, Hwang PM, Snyder SH: Localization of nitric oxide synthase indicating a neural role for nitric oxide. Nature 347:768–770, 1990
150. Kharazia VN, Schmidt HH, Weinberg RJ: Type I nitric oxide synthase fully accounts for NADPH-diaphorase in rat striatum, but not cortex. Neuroscience 62:983–987, 1994
151. Izuta M, Clavier N, Kirsch JR, Traystman RJ: Cerebral blood flow during inhibition of brain nitric oxide synthase activity in normal, hypertensive, and stroke-prone rats. Stroke 26:1079–1085, 1995
152. Garthwaite J, Garthwaite G, Palmer RM, Moncada S: NMDA receptor activation induces nitric oxide synthesis from arginine in rat brain slices. Eur J Pharmacol 172:413–416, 1989
153. Gendelman HE, Genis P, Jett M, Zhai QH, Nottet HS: An experimental model system for HIV-1-induced brain injury. Adv Neuroimmunol 4: 189–193, 1994
154. Kozniewska E, Roberts TP, Tsuura M, Mintorovitch J et al: NG-nitro-L-arginine delays the development of brain injury during focal ischemia in rats. Stroke 26:282–289, 1995
155. Sakashita N, Ando Y, Yonehara T, Tanaka Y et al: Role of superoxide dismutase and nitric oxide on the interaction between brain and systemic circulation during brain ischemia. Biochim Biomed Acta 1227:67–73, 1994
156. Nishikawa T, Kirsch JR, Koeshler RC, Miyabe M, Traystman RJ: Nitric oxide synthase inhibition reduces caudate injury following transient focal ischemia in cats. Stroke 25:877–885, 1994

157. Cazevieille C, Muller A, Meynier F, Bonne C: Superoxide and nitric oxide cooperation in hypoxia/reoxygenation-induced neuron injury. Free Radic Biology Med 14:389–395, 1993

158. Butler J, Rocker GM, Westaby S: Inflammatory response to cardiopulmonary bypass. Ann Thorac Surg 55:552–559, 1993

159. Moat NE, Shore DF, Evans TW: Organ dysfunction and cardiopulmonary bypass: The role of complement and complement regulatory proteins. Eur J Cardiothorac Surg 7:563–573, 1993

160. Seghaye MC, Duchateau J, Grabitz RG, Faymonville ML: Complement activation during cardiopulmonary bypass in infants and children: Relation to postoperative multiple system organ failure. J Thorac Cardiovasc Surg 106:978–987, 1993

161. Rinder CS, Gaal D, Student LA, Smith BR: Platelet-leukocyte activation and modulation of adhesion receptors in pediatric patients with congenital heart disease undergoing cardiopulmonary bypass. J Thorac Cardiovasc Surg 107:280–288, 1994

162. Plotz FB, van Oeveren W, Bartlett RH, Wildevuur CRH: Blood activation during neonatal extracorporeal life support. J Thorac Cardiovasc Surg 105:823–832, 1993

163. Kawamura T, Wakusawa R, Okada K, Inada S: Elevation of cytokines during open heart surgery with cardiopulmonary bypass: Participation of interleukin 8 and 6 in reperfusion injury. Can J Anaesth 40:1016–1021, 1993

164. Wachtfogel YT, Kucich U, Hames HL et al: Human plasma kallikrein releases neutrophil elastase during blood coagulation. J Clin Invest 72: 1672–1677, 1983

165. Wachtfogel YT, Pixley RA, Kucich U et al: Purified plasma factor XIIa aggregates human neutrophils and causes degranulation. Blood 67: 1731–1737, 1986

166. Skaryak LA, Kirshbom PM, DiBernardo LR, Kern FH et al: Modified ultrafiltration improves cerebral metabolic recovery after circulatory arrest. J Thorac Cardiovasc Surg 109:744–751, 1995

167. Feuerstein GZ, Liu T, Barone FC: Cytokines, inflammation, and brain injury: Role of tumor necrosis factor-α. Cerebrovasc Brain Metab Rev 6: 341–360, 1994

168. Saitoh T, Masliah E, Jim L-W, Cole GM et al: Protein kinases and phosphorylation in neurologic disorders and cell death. Lab Invest 64: 596–616, 1991

169. Sarafian TA, Bredesen DE: Is apoptosis mediated by reactive oxygen species? Free Radic Res Commun 21:1–8, 1994

170. Itoh N, Yonehara S, Ishii A, Yonehara M et al: The polypeptide encoded by the cDNA for human cell surface antigen Fas can mediate apoptosis. Cell 66:233–243, 1991

171. Yonehara S, Ishii A, Yonehara M: A cell-killing monoclonal antibody (anti-Fas) to a cell surface antigen co-downregulated with the receptor of tumor necrosis factor. J Exp Med 169:1747–1756, 1989

172. Miyawaki T, Uehara T, Nibu R, Tsuji T et al: Differential expression of apoptosis-related Fas antigen on lymphocyte subpopulations in human peripheral blood. J Immunol 149:3753–3758, 1992

173. Tanaka M, Ito H, Adachi S, Akimoto H et al: Hypoxia induces apoptosis with enhanced expression of Fas antigen messenger RNA in cultured neonatal rat cardiomyocytes. Circ Res 75:426–433, 1994

174. Demczuk S, Levy A, Aubry M, Croquette MF et al: Excess of deletions of maternal original in the DiGeorge/velo-cardio-facial syndromes: A study of 22 new patients and review of the literature. Hum Genet 96: 9–13, 1995
175. Menasche P, Peynet J, Lariviere J, Tronc F et al: Does normothermia during cardiopulmonary bypass increase neutrophil-endothelium interactions? Circulation 90(part 2):II275–II279, 1994
176. Nagle WA, Soloff BL, Moss AJ Jr, Henle KJ: Cultured Chinese hamster cells undergo apoptosis after exposure to cold but nonfreezing temperatures. Cryobiology 27:439–451, 1990

Susan C. Nicolson
James M. Steven
David R. Jobes

6 | Univentricular Heart: Staging through the Fontan Operation

Long-term survival of a newborn whose heart has only one functional ventricle depends upon a reduction in ventricular volume and pressure work to that of a normal systemic ventricle while perfusing the body with fully oxygenated blood. Because such an arrangement does not exist in nature, this strategy requires the surgical creation of a circulation in which the ventricle pumps fully saturated blood only to the systemic circulation, and the systemic venous return passes through the pulmonary vascular bed without the aid of a pumping chamber (i.e., systemic and pulmonary circuits connected in "series"). Contemporary methods to achieve these goals represent the culmination of the pioneering work of Glenn,[1] Fontan and Baudet,[2] and Kreutzer et al.[3] The physiologically high pulmonary vascular resistance of the neonate and young infant precludes sufficient pulmonary blood flow in the absence of a cardiac pump, thereby preventing successful execution of this series configuration early in life. In order to overcome the normal neonatal pulmonary vascular resistance, the great vessels must arise directly from the ventricle or be connected at the arterial level; the ventricle thus pumps blood directly to both systemic and pulmonary circulations in a "parallel" configuration.

At this young age, measures directed at preservation of ventricular function while permitting normal pulmonary vascular maturation to occur comprise the goals of palliative surgery. Ventricular preser-

Perioperative Management of the Patient with Congenital Heart Disease, edited by William J. Greeley. Williams & Wilkins, Baltimore © 1996.

vation is generally optimal when the pressure and volume work performed are minimized. Complete relief of any outflow tract and valvar or aortic obstruction assures minimal pressure work, while the volume work a single ventricle performs in a parallel configuration corresponds to the sum of systemic (Qs) and pulmonary (Qp) blood flows. Optimal pulmonary to systemic flow ratio (Qp:Qs) represents a compromise of cost and benefits. Progressive increases in Qp:Qs provide higher systemic oxygen saturation at the cost of greater volume work. Because most univentricular hearts can accommodate twice normal volume output without debilitating heart failure, and relatively normal growth and development can occur with systemic saturation in that range (70 to 80%), we strive for a Qp:Qs ratio near 1. This physiology must be considered palliative because of the morbidity from resulting chronic volume overload of the ventricle and hypoxemia from intracardiac mixing of systemic venous and pulmonary venous blood.

Once the pulmonary vascular resistance has fallen to normal, consideration should be given to prompt separation of the circulations. The increase in the ventricle's muscle mass during the requisite period of increased volume work not infrequently results in "relative" hypertrophy and diastolic dysfunction when end-diastolic volume acutely falls as a result of direct conversion from a parallel to a series circuit.[4,5] In the absence of a pulmonary pump, these changes in diastolic function or compliance may exert a deleterious effect on pulmonary blood flow and, hence, systemic cardiac output. Accomplishing the conversion to a series circulation via two procedures permits the volume load of the single ventricle to be reduced to normal while minimizing the impact of rapid change in ventricular geometry on cardiac output.[6,7] Once the ventricle has accommodated to a lower end-diastolic volume with remodeling and increased compliance, the series configuration can be completed. This management strategy has evolved over the last two decades and has been successfully applied to the entire spectrum of congenital cardiac malformations with a single ventricle.

NEWBORN PERIOD TO FIRST STAGE OF THE FONTAN PROCEDURE

Regardless of the precise anatomical configuration (e.g., tricuspid atresia (TA), hypoplastic left heart syndrome (HLHS), double outlet ventricle, etc.), pulmonary blood flow in a neonate with a univentricular heart malformation must be derived in parallel with the systemic circulation to take advantage of the higher driving pressure necessary to overcome high pulmonary vascular resistance. When surgical intervention is required in these neonates, it most commonly consists of procedures that establish or regulate the arterial level communications in order to assure pulmonary and systemic blood flow in nearly equal proportions (e.g., shunt, band, or complex reconstructions as in Norwood procedure). If the vascular anatomy is properly configured to achieve a Qp:Qs of unity, pulmonary blood flow will be adequate for systemic oxygen delivery, resulting in normal growth and development while limiting the volume work imposed on the ventricle to twice normal.

In addition, the conditions necessary to permit the normal maturational decline in pulmonary vascular resistance merit particular attention, usually by assuring unobstructed pulmonary venous return, then limiting the blood pressure and flow to which the pulmonary circulation is exposed to values that approach normal. Structurally limited pulmonary flow coupled with unobstructed pulmonary venous drainage will result in the pulmonary vascular resistance falling over a time course similar to other newborns.

Direct conversion from a parallel to series circulation in the first 12 to 18 months of life in a subset of children (HLHS: Norwood procedure) resulted in a high operative mortality.[8-10] The most common cause of early death was low cardiac output associated with tachycardia, low systolic and diastolic arterial blood pressure, and high ventricular end-diastolic and pulmonary artery pressures. Most children with low cardiac output in the immediate postoperative period demonstrated echocardiographic evidence of an abrupt change in ventricular geometry that followed the acute reduction in the volume load imposed on the single ventricle.[11] When compared to the preoperative state, these studies revealed a small, thick-walled cavity with a low end-diastolic volume. Although systolic shortening appeared normal, the ventricular compliance was diminished by hemodynamic assessment. An anatomical consequence of this sudden relief of volume work is an apparent increase in wall thickness because muscle mass does not thin as rapidly as end-diastolic volume diminishes. The physiological result is impaired diastolic function of the ventricle leading to increased end-diastolic pressure.[5] The resultant increase in pulmonary venous pressure impedes pulmonary blood flow, thereby reducing systemic output. Retrospective analysis of the data available preoperatively proved insufficient to predict those children who would develop a physiologically important reduction of ventricular compliance associated with rapid contraction of end-diastolic volume following creation of a series circulation. In many centers, observations supported the concept that children following Fontan operation in whom a residual right-to-left shunt persisted as a result of baffle leaks or unrecognized anomalies of systemic venous return demon-strated reduced morbidity and mortality.[12] This led to the concept of staging the conversion.

FIRST STAGE: HEMI-FONTAN OR BIDIRECTIONAL GLENN PROCEDURE

Goals

The principal objectives of the first component of a staged Fontan sequence are to reduce the ventricular volume load to normal and allow myocardial remodeling to occur at a lower end-diastolic volume without a substantially deleterious impact on cardiac output. In fact, a staged approach to the Fontan procedure permits reduction in ven-tricular volume demand to that of a normal ventricle earlier in life (i.e., 6 months) than direct (one-stage) Fontan surgery ever allowed. Two options have gained acceptance as the first step of a staged con-version; bidirectional Glenn operation[7,13] or hemi-Fontan.[6,10] In this type of Glenn procedure, the superior vena cava is divided and anas-tomosed to the undivided pulmonary arteries creating bidirectional cavopulmonary blood flow. This source of pulmonary blood flow may be exclusive if previous shunts are ligated or additive if they are not occluded. When previous sources of pulmonary blood flow are oc-cluded, it provides a physiological benefit similar to that of the hemi-Fontan procedure and can be performed without cardiopulmonary bypass.

During the hemi-Fontan procedure all systemic to pulmonary ar-tery shunts are ligated, and pulmonary blood flow is achieved exclu-sively via a superior vena cava to pulmonary artery anastomosis.[6,10] Although a subtle distinction, it guarantees that the volume work im-posed on the ventricle is equivalent to that of a normal ventricle sup-plying only the systemic circulation (Qs). In addition, the use of cardiopulmonary bypass enables simultaneous correction of any co-existing anatomical risk factors (e.g., restrictive interatrial communi-cation, pulmonary artery deformities, AV valve regurgitation, aortic arch obstruction). The hemi-Fontan operation also preserves the nor-mal relationship of the superior vena cava to right atrium, simplifying the subsequent procedure.

Following either intervention hypoxemia persists. Over the en-suing several months the ratio of ventricular mass to volume will normalize, and consideration can be given to baffling the inferior vena cava blood into the superior vena cava-pulmonary artery anastomosis, thereby completing separation of the circuits. This eliminates hypoxemia and reduces the potential for paradoxical emboli and the formation of pulmonary arteriovenous malformations, the latter having been associated with Glenn-type reconstructions. While HLHS represents the most common univentricular heart malformation, these findings are not confined to infants with that anatomical diagnosis. Rather, these physiological principles apply to all univentricular hearts, as the pathophysiological consequences of direct (one-stage) Fontan procedures have been observed across a spectrum of anatomical variants. Failure to predict those who will manifest this pathophysiology after direct conversion coupled with the lethal consequences of the same constitutes a compelling argument for staging all patients. Nevertheless, some controversy still persists with respect to the merits of other methods designed to provide significant right-to-left shunts (e.g., large baffle fenestrations) as a means of sustaining cardiac output during changes in ventricular compliance, particularly in older patients.[14,15]

Preoperative Considerations

Routine preanesthetic evaluation is performed, and the results of the hemodynamic profile including cardiac catheterization and echocardiogram are reviewed. Features affecting "passive" blood flow through the pulmonary circulation merit particular attention. They include pulmonary vascular resistance, AV valve function, and the end-diastolic pressure in the ventricle. Significant pathophysiology in any of these elements will increase the pulmonary artery or superior vena cava pressure necessary to drive flow through the pulmonary circulation. As such, postoperative pulmonary artery pressure represents a reasonably sensitive index integrating all the physiological factors important to well-being after hemi-Fontan or Fontan procedures. In a series of 129 patients undergoing bidirectional Glenn operation, Alejos and colleagues demonstrated significantly lower mortality when postoperative pulmonary artery pressure remained under 18 mm Hg (4 vs 20%).[16] Using the predicted change in pulmonary blood flow that accompanies this operation, one can estimate postoperative pulmonary artery pressure (Fig. 6–1). For example, if the preoperative Qp:Qs is unity, then pulmonary blood flow will be reduced approximately by half following this procedure, because the superior vena cava typically drains structures that receive 45% of the cardiac output. Assuming constant pulmonary vascular resistance, the gradient from pulmonary artery to pulmonary veins (ΔP) will likewise be halved. Adding ΔP to left atrial pressure provides an estimate of postoperative pulmonary artery pressure. These estimates do not incorporate the alterations in ventricular compliance that often accompany acute

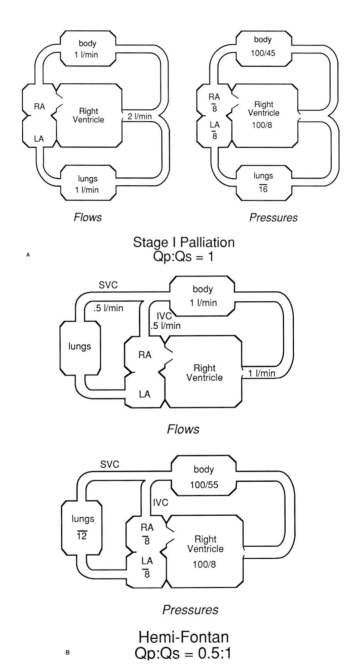

FIGURE 6–1. Schematic representation of pressures and flows in a representative example of a univentricular heart before and after hemi-Fontan (*A* and *B*, respectively). Flows in panel *A* reflect the volume load imposed by a Qp:Qs of 1 in a parallel circulation. Panel *B* illustrates the changes expected in the con-

reduction in the ventricular volume load. Physiological features indicating extraordinary ventricular volume or pressure loads pre-operatively might predispose the ventricle to even greater diastolic dysfunction postoperatively (e.g., Qp:Qs substantially above unity or aortic arch obstruction).

Physiological Consequences

Two important physiological changes distinguish the child following superior vena cava-pulmonary artery connection: systemic cardiac output does not exhibit either a direct or inverse dependence on pulmonary blood flow, and the driving force propelling blood through the lung is substantially reduced. When the systemic and pulmonary circulations are connected in parallel, reductions in pulmonary vascular resistance result in increased pulmonary blood flow, diverting flow from the systemic circulation and increasing the cardiac output placed upon the ventricle in order to satisfy systemic metabolical requirements. At a critical threshold, the ventricle can increase its output no further, and systemic flow falls. In this extreme, cardiac output and pulmonary blood flow are inversely related. Occluding the arterial communications between systemic and pulmonary circuits eliminates the conditions under which reduction in pulmonary vascular resistance increases the volume work on the ventricle. After a hemi-Fontan procedure, children do not exhibit the critical relationship that follows a complete Fontan operation in which pulmonary blood flow exclusively determines systemic output. When anatomical or physiological barriers impede pulmonary blood flow after a hemi-Fontan, inferior vena cava flow acts to preserve ventricular filling and systemic output. Although systemic output is buffered from changes in pulmonary blood flow, systemic oxygenation is not. Rather than a direct connection with the systemic arterial circulation, pulmonary blood flow is propelled by a moderate increase in systemic venous pressure. Thus, subtle increases in pulmonary vascular resistance will reduce pulmonary blood flow and, consequently, the proportion of oxygenated venous return to the atrium with resulting decrease in systemic arterial saturation.

Although output requirements placed on the single ventricle are reduced to normal, the systemic saturation is virtually unchanged.

---

version to hemi-Fontan. Cardiac output falls to that level necessary to perfuse only the body. Assuming constant pulmonary vascular resistance, the pressure gradient across the lungs falls in proportion to the reduction in flow (see text for calculation method).

Pulmonary blood flow arises exclusively from superior vena cava drainage. Saturated pulmonary venous blood mixes in the common atrium with nearly an equal quantity of desaturated blood draining from the inferior vena cava resulting in an expected systemic arterial oxygen saturation between 80 and 85%. Pulmonary blood flow and hence systemic arterial oxygenation is critically dependent on the interrelationship of pulmonary vascular resistance, superior vena cava pressure (which equals pulmonary artery pressure), and pulmonary venous pressure. At a constant pulmonary vascular resistance, the pulmonary pressure gradient (Δ = pulmonary artery − pulmonary venous pressure) determines pulmonary blood flow. Similarly, pulmonary vascular resistance will determine pulmonary blood flow if the ΔP is constant. Increased pulmonary venous pressure usually arises from atrioventricular valve dysfunction or impaired ventricular diastolic function, whereas decreased superior vena cava pressure indicates hypovolemia.

Postoperative Considerations

Apart from the usual considerations following reconstructive cardiac surgery in young infants, patients following the hemi-Fontan procedure merit particular attention to any factors that promote passive pulmonary blood flow.

Ventilation and Oxygenation

Balancing carbon dioxide elimination against the increased peak or mean airway pressure necessary to achieve that degree of ventilation represents the fundamental quandary in the ventilatory manipulation of pulmonary vascular resistance. Excessive airway pressure transmitted to the intraacinar vessels diverts blood away from the pulmonary vascular bed, thereby exacerbating hypoxemia. The pattern of controlled ventilation that most reliably provides hypocapnia while minimizing transmitted airway pressure entails moderately large tidal volumes (e.g., preset values between 25 and 30 ml/kg, delivered 15 to 20 ml/kg), slow respiratory rates (16 to 20 breaths/min), and short inspiratory (I) and long expiratory (E) time (I:E of 1:3 to 1:4). A reduction in pulmonary vascular resistance will not impose a volume load on the ventricle because the pulmonary and systemic arterial circulations are no longer connected in parallel. The analysis of significant hypoxemia ($PaO_2 < 30$ mm Hg) should encompass anatomical or technical issues that include the superior vena cava-pulmonary artery anastomosis and previously unrecognized venous communications between the upper body and the heart (e.g., left superior vena cava, azygous vein to inferior vena cava). Functional issues to be considered include increased pulmonary vascular resistance from ineffective or excessive ventilation, hypothermia and/or acidemia, as well as insufficient pulmonary artery driving pressure due to inadequate circulating volume.

Intravascular Volume

The maintenance of sufficient intravascular volume assumes tremendous importance in order to provide an adequate pressure gradient to promote pulmonary blood flow. Volume requirements are guided by heart rate, and atrial, pulmonary artery, and systemic arterial pressures. Direct pressure measurements in the superior vena cava-pulmonary artery and atrium can be used to infer changes in pulmonary vascular resistance and diastolic function of the ventricle.

Pharmacological Intervention

Inotropes

In the absence of intraoperative myocardial injury, ventricular performance after the hemi-Fontan procedure typically reflects the benefit of a reduced volume output requirement. Doppler studies indicate that "passive" pulmonary blood flow (i.e., resulting from nonphasic pressure gradients rather than a pump) occurs disproportionately during diastole.[17] Therefore, primary considerations in selecting the characteristics of an inotropic agent include minimal tachycardia and limited α-adrenergic agonism in order to avoid increased pulmonary vascular resistance. Although dopamine or dobutamine in doses under 5 μg/kg/minute generally meets these objectives, amrinone also possesses the desired characteristics. While isoproterenol may lower pulmonary vascular resistance, its impact on heart rate limits its utility. Epinephrine exerts a negative impact on pulmonary vascular resistance and heart rate at doses necessary to achieve inotropy, exceeding that of dopamine or dobutamine.

Afterload-Reducing Agents

Pharmacological reduction in systemic vascular resistance has favorably influenced cardiac output in a selected group of infants after the hemi-Fontan procedure. These infants typically exhibit a severely dilated ventricle preoperatively, due to primary myocardial disease or, more commonly, as a result of the excessive volume load imposed by a high Qp:Qs or AV valve insufficiency. They will characteristically exhibit diminished peripheral perfusion as evidenced by reduced peripheral pulses, capillary refill, and skin temperature in association with normal or elevated core temperature. Sodium nitroprusside (0.5 to 5 μg/kg/min) has proven useful in providing rapid onset, efficacy, and titratable effects. Vasodilatation usually increases venous capacitance further, necessitating administration of supplemental fluid.

In many respects, the child with a hemi-Fontan procedure has the most resilient physiology of the staged reconstructive repairs for the univentricular heart. The ventricle no longer bears the increased volume load, and yet the systemic cardiac output is not critically dependent on pulmonary blood flow. If pulmonary blood flow declines, return from the inferior vena cava serves to maintain ventricular preload and thus preserves cardiac output. Although qualitatively similar ventricular diastolic changes seen after the primary Fontan procedure may occur, the manifestations are limited to a "superior vena cava (SVC) syndrome" rather than low cardiac output, and quantitative reductions in ventricular volume and increases in wall thickness are smaller.[18] Two-dimensional echocardiography in 19 infants in the early postoperative period following a hemi-Fontan or primary (one-stage) Fontan procedure showed an average reduction in ventricular end-diastolic dimensions of 24 vs 46% and a concomitant increase in ventricular wall thickness of 9 vs 43%, respectively.

SECOND STAGE: COMPLETION FONTAN PROCEDURE

Preoperative Considerations

Precise timing of the completion Fontan requires a judgment weighing several offsetting considerations, each of which is incompletely understood. At a minimum, the interval between stages must permit restoration of optimal ventricular compliance at its new end-diastolic dimension. In the absence of a diagnostic tool sufficiently sensitive or specific to evaluate this process, we have arbitrarily established a minimal interval of 6 months. Despite its hemodynamic resilience, after the hemi-Fontan operation the resultant anatomy and physiology of infants do pose some risks that may prove compelling reasons not to extend the interval inordinately. These infants are subject to the risks of paradoxical emboli returning via the inferior vena cava as well as the physiological consequences of hypoxemia that typically accelerate with age. In addition, diversion of inferior vena cava blood away from the pulmonary circulation predisposes to the development of pulmonary arteriovenous malformations that presumably would otherwise be inhibited by a factor elaborated in the liver. While initially a recognized sequela of Glenn shunts,[19] this phenomenon has been observed in a few infants and children following the initial component of a staged Fontan operation.

Anatomical and hemodynamic assessment is obtained and interpreted in light of the expected changes that result from a Fontan operation. A constant physiological feature after a Fontan procedure is elevation of the systemic venous pressure (systemic venous pressure = pulmonary artery pressure) to the level necessary to promote adequate pulmonary blood flow to support cardiac output. Catheterization data prior to the Fontan procedure enable an estimate of postoperative hemodynamics. With a systemic saturation between 80 and 85% suggesting typical pulmonary blood flow after hemi-Fontan (i.e., Qp:Qs of 0.5:1), completion of the Fontan operation should nearly double pulmonary blood flow, thus doubling the pressure gradient from the pulmonary artery to the pulmonary veins. An approximation of the postoperative pulmonary artery pressure is obtained by adding the predicted pulmonary artery to pulmonary vein gradient to the left atrial pressure.

Postoperative Considerations

Morbidity and mortality after Fontan's operation usually relate to the systemic venous pressure necessary to provide sufficient pulmonary blood to enable satisfactory cardiac output. In a manner analogous to that after the hemi-Fontan procedure, the determinants of eventual systemic venous pressure include: 1) pulmonary vascular resistance, encompassing both microcirculatory physiology as well as mechanical obstruction to pulmonary artery or pulmonary venous flow, 2) ventricular compliance as reflected by the end-diastolic pressure in the ventricle, and 3) atrioventricular valve function.

A number of options exist as a means of ensuring satisfactory cardiac output while diminishing the consequences of elevated systemic venous pressure. As a means of limiting morbidity and mortality in the event that alterations in PVR or ventricular compliance impede pulmonary blood flow, "partial" or "fenestrated" Fontan procedures allow deliberate right-to-left shunting of blood at the atrial level.[12,14,15] This beneficial effect on cardiac output is realized at the expense of a physiologically acceptable reduction in systemic arterial oxygen saturation.

Ventilation and Oxygenation

The fundamental principles of ventilation following complete Fontan operation are identical to those described after the first stage; however, the impact of ineffective or deleterious patterns of ventilation is more clandestine. Ventilatory management that promotes elevated pulmonary vascular resistance will impede pulmonary blood flow. Hypoxemia, the principal sign of diminished pulmonary blood flow following hemi-Fontan, is obvious and reliably quantified. However, the principal consequence of diminished pulmonary blood flow following the Fontan operation, low cardiac output, is both insidious and ultimately more malignant. In the operating room, the signs are confined to systemic hypotension, tachycardia, and widening pulmonary arterial-atrial pressure gradient. Metabolical acidemia develops late in the course of low cardiac output. Elevated pulmonary vascular resistance with decreased pulmonary blood flow can be associated with excessive intrathoracic pressure. Disconnecting the child from the breathing circuit will result in a prompt decline in pulmonary artery pressure and an increase in systemic arterial pressure. Alternative explanations for an elevated pulmonary vascular resistance include: inadequate functional residual capacity, increased alveolar Pco_2, low alveolar Po_2, hypothermia, and pleural accumulations (e.g., blood, gas, or serous effusion).

Doppler interrogation confirms that conventional mechanical positive pressure ventilation exerts a negative impact on the velocity or even the direction of pulmonary blood flow.[20] Thus, the ventilatory pattern should be designed to maintain the lungs expanded to normal functional residual capacity at end-exhalation while using the minimal peak and mean airway pressure necessary to achieve satisfactory gas exchange. After Fontan's operation most children can be managed with conventional positive pressure ventilation without signs of a deleterious effect on cardiac output. In patients requiring substantially increased pulmonary artery pressure to promote adequate pulmonary blood flow (e.g., elevated pulmonary vascular resistance or ventricular dysfunction with elevated ventricular end-diastolic pressure), the increase in mean airway pressure may result in a clinically important reduction in an already marginal systemic output. High-frequency jet ventilation offers a major advantage over conventional mechanical ventilation in its ability to provide equivalent alveolar P_{CO_2} and P_{O_2} at reduced mean airway pressure. Meliones and colleagues conducted a cross-over study comparing conventional ventilation with high-frequency jet ventilation in 13 children (0.9 to 8.5 yr) during the early postoperative period following Fontan's operation.[21] Jet ventilation resulted in a 50% reduction in mean airway pressure, a 59% reduction in pulmonary vascular resistance, and a 25% increase in cardiac index.

Spontaneous ventilation is particularly desirable because Doppler-based studies have demonstrated an associated significant increase in pulmonary blood flow (up to 64%).[20] If signs of respiratory or cardiovascular embarrassment occur, positive pressure ventilatory support is reinstituted. A beneficial effect on hemodynamics nearly always results despite incontrovertible evidence that mechanical ventilation can impede pulmonary blood flow. Possible explanations include: 1) pulmonary vascular resistance increases as alveolar P_{CO_2} rises even slightly; 2) ventricular diastolic function deteriorates in relation to the increased metabolical demand imposed by spontaneous ventilation; or 3) a deleterious effect on either ventricular compliance or pulmonary vascular resistance may result from release of endogenous catecholamines.

Intravascular Volume

The manipulation of intravascular volume and hence pulmonary artery pressure represents the other variable that exerts a direct impact on pulmonary blood flow. Because the elevated venous pressure is now present throughout the entire body, the increased vascular capacitance may exceed that seen following the first stage. These children require constant vigilance to recognize the subtle signs of hypovolemia and diminished systemic output. Tachycardia represents one of the earliest indicators of inadequate cardiac filling in these children, whether due to hypovolemia or an impediment to pulmonary blood flow. An elevated gradient between core and distal extremity temperature, particularly with core hyperpyrexia, provides supporting evidence of diminished peripheral blood flow. While systemic venous and atrial pressures provide irreplaceable information, they are not ultimately sensitive or specific determinants of intravascular volume inasmuch as they reflect the dynamic product of vascular tone and diastolic ventricular function as well. Hypotension and acidemia represent late findings of inadequate systemic flow.

Pharmacological Support

Inotropes

Echocardiographic evaluation may provide information that helps direct further therapy in the presence of hypotension, despite maximal intravascular volume supplementation, or persistent signs of inadequate systemic perfusion despite vasodilators. Assessment of ventricular volume constitutes the most valuable echocardiographic information apart from severe AV valve insufficiency or anatomical obstructions amenable to surgical therapy. A ventricle dilated from acquired myocardial disease or AV valve insufficiency has the potential to respond favorably to inotropic agents. A ventricle that is hypertrophic and hypercontractile with poor diastolic relaxation and a small volume is far less common after a staged Fontan than after a primary Fontan procedure. Reduced ventricular compliance leads to elevated end-diastolic pressure which serves to impede pulmonary blood flow and ultimately compromise ventricular output. Because the primary functional problem of these small ventricles resides in diastole rather than systole, inotropic agents are notoriously ineffective at achieving more than short-term elevations in systemic arterial pressure.

Afterload Reducing Agents

When subtle signs of insufficient systemic output persist after augmenting intravascular volume, systemic vasodilatation often ameliorates the findings. Sodium nitroprusside, titrated to the desired effect, has proven particularly efficacious.

Outcome after the Fontan Operation

Survival

Staged Fontan reconstruction has been associated with significant reduction in morbidity and mortality. Operative mortality at the Children's Hospital of Philadelphia is well below 5% for each stage. Mortality as a result of the hemi-Fontan procedure appears to increase when that procedure is performed on infants under 4 months of age. Whether this incremental risk reflects a degree of maturation that is incompatible with hemi-Fontan physiology or simply a manifestation of the selected population that requires intervention that early (e.g., uncontrollable heart failure or debilitating hypoxemia) remains uncertain.

Arrhythmias

Arrhythmias may complicate the early and late course after the Fontan operation. Atrial tachyarrhythmias, such as flutter, tend to be associated with unsatisfactory hemodynamics early in the postoperative period but are better tolerated beyond 1 month.[22] Atrial tachyarrhythmias seem to be associated more commonly with surgical techniques that leave a substantial portion of atrial tissue exposed to systemic venous pressure.[23]

Effusions

Pleural and pericardial effusions can have deleterious effects on pulmonary vascular resistance and ventricular compliance, respectively, and represent a significant source of morbidity after the Fontan operation. Although many have attempted to define the mechanism(s) by which they form, the etiology remains elusive. A biochemical basis was sought by Stewart et al. who measured plasma vasopressin and atrial natriuretic factor (ANF) in 19 children before, during, and after the Fontan procedure.[24] Vasopressin and ANF levels were higher preoperatively and increased more after surgery in Fontan patients compared to 12 control patients with two ventricles undergoing cardiac procedures requiring bypass. Vasopressin levels remained elevated longer in patients undergoing Fontan and were highest in children with the most severe fluid retention. The authors postulate that increased vasopressin and ANF could act synergistically to result in the development of effusion when ANF-induced capillary transudation is combined with vasopressin-induced antidiuresis.

The incidence and the magnitude of effusions after the first stage are dramatically lower, even when the pulmonary artery pressure is similar. One theory links elevated hepatic venous pressure after the Fontan operation with the propensity to develop effusions. A number of Fontan procedures have been performed where one or two of the hepatic veins were intentionally excluded from the inferior vena cava-pulmonary artery baffle, enabling them to drain directly into the lower pressure of the atrium. Our experience demonstrated a substantial reduction in the incidence of clinically significant thoracic effusions with partial hepatic vein exclusion (10 vs 54%), but progressive right-to-left shunts via the hepatic circulation resulted in hypoxemia necessitating reinclusion of the hepatic veins in a significant proportion of these children. Baffle fenestration has also afforded a beneficial impact on the development of serous effusions.[25]

Gastrointestinal System

Passive congestion of the liver is a virtually ubiquitous finding after the Fontan operation. Although some elevation in serum concentration of hepatic enzymes often accompanies this congestion, impaired hepatosynthetic function or cholestasis rarely occurs. In a small subpopulation, the consequences of Fontan physiology may induce a protein-losing enteropathy (PLE). While intuitive reasoning might logically lead one to indict systemic venous hypertension as the primary cause, in fact, hemodynamic studies have repeatedly failed to corroborate any quantifiable relationship between caval pressure and PLE. This condition reflects the combined effects of gastrointestinal congestion, impaired absorption, and reduced lymphatic drainage. This pathophysiology further aggravates existing hypoalbuminemia and contributes to peripheral edema. When refractory to medical management, surgical baffle fenestration has proven successful in ameliorating PLE in a small series of patients.[26]

FURTHER INTERVENTIONS FOLLOWING FONTAN

Fenestrated Fontan procedures are designed to enable the interatrial communication to be closed later via a closed cardiac procedure or interventional catheterization. Transcatheter closure of the communication offers the advantage of a hemodynamic assessment of systemic venous pressure during test occlusion followed by permanent closure with a double-umbrella device.[14] Whether this procedure transpires early or late in the postoperative period depends on the child's hemodynamics and systemic oxygenation. Unfortunately, most centers without access to such devices must explore alternate strategies. Multiple (3) small fenestrations (2.7 mm) appear to offer the advantage of permitting early postoperative shunting, reducing the incidence of serous effusions, with the prospect of subsequent spontaneous closure in the majority of children.

Children and young adults who have undergone a Fontan operation merit careful follow-up and early intervention when pathophysiological processes develop that might threaten the performance of their single ventricle. Examples include AV valve dysfunction, arrhythmias, or progressive outflow tract obstruction (e.g., closing ventricular septal defect that provides flow to the aorta via an outlet chamber). Despite flawless care, some single ventricles will ultimately fail, necessitating heart replacement. The anesthetic management of children with compromised Fontan physiology demands consummate skill and caution as they are exquisitely sensitive to myocardial depressants, intravascular volume, and ventilatory manipulations.

CONCLUSIONS

In a 20-year multiinstitutional follow-up study of patients who had undergone the primary Fontan operation and exhibited a good early result, Fontan et al. reported a steady decline in heart function according to the New York Heart Classification such that 50% were class II 15 years postoperatively.[27] Actuarial survival declined from 92% at 1 month to 73% at 15 years. The continued decline in both functional result and survival caused Fontan to classify the procedure as palliative.

Many features in the management of children with univentricular hearts have changed in the quarter century since Fontan proposed his operation. A profound sensitivity to the importance of preservation of ventricular function has lead to earlier interventions designed to alleviate excessive loading conditions. Similarly, technical features of the operation that often resulted in significant late sequelae (e.g., valved venous conduits, huge hypertensive atria) have been substantially simplified or eliminated. No comparable long-term outcome data currently exist for patients undergoing a staged Fontan. Hopefully, this strategy in association with all the other evolutionary modifications will result in improved function and outcome inasmuch as the Fontan operation remains the only reconstructive option for the 5 to 10% of children with congenital heart disease born with a univentricular heart.

References

1. Glenn WWL: Circulatory bypass of the right heart. N Engl J Med 259: 117–120, 1958
2. Fontan F, Baudet E: Surgical repair of tricuspid atresia. Thorax 26:240–248, 1971

3. Kreutzer GO, Galindex E, Bono H: An operation for correction of tricuspid atresia. J Thorac Cardiovasc Surg 66:613–621, 1973
4. Penny DJ, Redington AN: Diastolic ventricular function after the Fontan operation. Am J Cardiol 69:974–975, 1992
5. Penny DJ, Lincoln C, Shore DR, Xiao HB, Rigby ML, Redington AN: The early response of the systemic ventricle during transition to the Fontan circulation: An acute cardiomyopathy? Cardiol Young 2:78–84, 1992
6. Douville EC, Sade RM, Fyfe DA: Hemi-Fontan operation in surgery for single ventricle: A preliminary report. Ann Thorac Surg 51:893–900, 1991
7. Lamberti JJ, Spicer RL, Waldman JD, Grehl TM, Thomson D, George L, Kirkpatrick SE, Mathewson JW: The bidirectional cavopulmonary shunt. J Thorac Cardiovasc Surg 100:22–30, 1990
8. Farrell PE Jr., Chang AC, Murdison KA, Baffa JM, Norwood WI, Murphy JD: Outcome and assessment after the modified Fontan procedure for hypoplastic left heart syndrome. Circulation 85:116–122, 1992
9. Bove EL: Transplantation after first-stage reconstruction for hypoplastic left heart syndrome. Ann Thorac Surg 52:701–707, 1991
10. Norwood WI, Murphy JD, Jacobs ML: Fontan procedure for hypoplastic left heart. Ann Thorac Surg 54:1025–1030, 1992
11. Chin AJ, Franklin WH, Andrews BA, Norwood WI: Changes in ventricular geometry early after Fontan operation. Ann Thorac Surg 56:1359–1365, 1993
12. Laks H: The partial Fontan procedure: A new concept and its clinical application. Circulation 82:1866–1867, 1990
13. Bridges ND, Jonas RA, Mayer JE, Flanagan MF, Keane JF, Castaneda AR: Bidirectional cavopulmonary anastomosis as interim palliation for high-risk Fontan candidates. Early results. Circulation 82:IV-170–IV-176, 1990
14. Bridges ND, Lock JE, Castaneda AR: Baffle fenestration with subsequent transcatheter closure. Modification of the Fontan operation for patients at increased risk. Circulation 82:1681–1689, 1990
15. Laks H, Pearl JM, Haas GS, Drinkwater DC, Milgalter E, Jarmakani JM, Isabel-Jones J, George BL, Williams RG: Partial Fontan: Advantages of an adjustable interatrial communication. Ann Thorac Surg 52:1084–1095, 1991
16. Alejos JC, Williams RG, Jarmakani JM, Galindo AJ, Isabel-Jones JB, Drinkwater D, Laks H, Kaplan S: Factors influencing survival in patients undergoing the bidirectional Glenn anastomosis. Am J Cardiol 75:1048–1050, 1995
17. Frommelt PC, Snider AR, Meliones JN, Vermilion RP: Doppler assessment of pulmonary artery flow patterns and ventricular function after the Fontan operation. Am J Cardiol 68:1211–1215, 1991
18. Rychik J, Jacobs ML, Norwood WI: Acute changes in left ventricular geometry after volume reduction operation. Ann Thorac Surg, in press, 1996
19. McFaul RC, Tajik AJ, Mair DD, Danielson GK, Seward JB: Development of pulmonary arteriovenous shunt after superior vena cava-right pulmonary artery (Glenn) anastomosis. Report of four cases. Circulation 55:212–216, 1977
20. Penny DJ, Redington AN: Doppler echocardiographic evaluation of pulmonary blood flow after the Fontan operation: The role of the lungs. Br Heart J 66:372–374, 1991
21. Meliones JN, Bove EL, Dekeon MK, Custer JR, Moler FW, Callow LR, Wilton NC, Rosen DB: High-frequency jet ventilation improves cardiac

function after the Fontan procedure. Circulation 84(suppl III):III-364–III-368, 1991

22. Gewillig M, Wyse RK, de Leval MR, Deanfield JE: Early and late arrhythmias after the Fontan operation: Predisposing factors and clinical consequences. Br Heart J 67:72–79, 1992

23. Balaji S, Gewillig M, Bull C, de Leval MR, Deanfield JE: Arrhythmias after the Fontan procedure. Comparison of total cavopulmonary connection and atriopulmonary connection. Circulation 84:III-162–III-167, 1991

24. Stewart JM, Gewitz MH, Clark BJ, Seligman KP, Romano A, Zeballos GA, Chang AC, Murdison KA, Woolf PK, Norwood WI: The role of vasopressin and atrial natriuretic factor in postoperative fluid retention after the Fontan procedure. J Thorac Cardiovasc Surg 102:821–829, 1991

25. Mayer JE, Bridges ND, Lock JE, Hanley FL, Jonas RA, Castaneda AR: Factors associated with marked reduction in mortality for Fontan operations in patients with single ventricle. J Thorac Cardiovasc Surg 103:444–451, 1992

26. Jacobs ML, Rychik J, Byrum CJ, Norwood WI: Protein-losing enteropathy after Fontan: Resolution after baffle fenestration. Ann Thorac Surg, in press, 1996

27. Fontan F, Kirklin JW, Fernandez G, Costa F, Naftel DC, Tritto F, Blackstone EH: Outcome after a "perfect" Fontan operation. Circulation 81:1520–1536, 1990

Dolly D. Hansen
Nancy D. Bridges

Perioperative Interventional Catheterization: The Anesthesiologist and the Cardiologist

7

The use of cardiac catheterization as a diagnostic tool for patients with congenital heart disease was first reported in 1947 by Bing and co-workers. Although angiographic imaging remains essential in many instances for structures that are beyond the hilum of the lung and in patients in whom echocardiographic imaging is suboptimal due to poor acoustic windows, advances in noninvasive cardiac imaging that have occurred over the last 10 years have produced a shift in emphasis in the cardiac catheterization laboratory, such that invasive studies are now performed primarily to obtain hemodynamic information and/ or for the purpose of transcatheter intervention. Although diagnostic catherizations are generally performed with sedation administered by specially trained nurses, without direct involvement by the anesthesia department, there are some instances (for example, children with se- verely elevated pulmonary vascular resistance (PVR), with develop- mental delay, or with an abnormal airway) in which the participation of a cardiac anesthesiologist is extremely valuable. This chapter, how- ever, will focus on the anesthesiologist's involvement in perioperative cardiac catheterizations performed for the purpose of transcatheter intervention.

That a catheter could be used for vascular therapy was demon- strated in 1964[2] with the dilation of acquired peripheral vascular ste- nosis by graduated rigid dilators. However, the balloon atrial septos-

Perioperative Management of the Patient with Congenital Heart Disease, edited by William J. Greeley. Williams & Wilkins, Baltimore © 1996.

tomy developed by Rashkind and Miller, reported in 1966,[3] was the first pediatric and the first intracardiac transcatheter therapy. Any of the procedures in the interventionist's repertoire might be performed in the pre- or postoperative patient. This chapter will focus on those that are most commonly indicated in this setting: balloon atrial septostomy in the newborn; atrial septal defect (ASD) creation in the older child; coil embolization of unwanted vascular communications (aortopulmonary collaterals, venovenous collaterals, patent ductus arteriosus, and surgically created aortopulmonary shunts); pulmonary artery dilation or stenting; closure of postoperative residual ASDs; closure of muscular ventricular septal defects (VSDs); and radiofrequency (RF) ablation of abnormal conduction pathways in patients in whom postoperative atrial arrhythmias will be poorly tolerated.

THE ANESTHESIOLOGIST'S VIEW

The anesthetist, who provides anesthetic support for the catheterization laboratory must, in cooperation with the cardiologist, decide whether it is better for a patient to be sedated or to receive general anesthesia. However, in reality this is only an issue in the preoperative patient, as the patient who needs interventional catherization in the immediate postoperative period most often is critically ill, on inotropic support, sedated, intubated, and fully ventilated. In these patients control of ventilation and avoidance of pulmonary hypertensive crisis are important. One postoperative exception is the patient with retained or broken intracardiac monitoring lines, who may already have been extubated and who can be managed with conventional sedation.

Routine patient monitoring includes an electrocardiogram (ECG), blood pressure, arterial oxygen saturation, and temperature. End-tidal carbon dioxide pressure is monitored continuously, either with nasal prongs in the spontaneously breathing patient or via a side arm in the breathing circuit in anesthetized patients. Secure intravenous access is established to provide additional sedation or resuscitation. Once the cardiologist has arterial and venous catheters in place, beat-to-beat monitoring of the arterial pressure, measurements of filling pressure, and arterial blood-gas analysis are readily available.

One problem that has emerged with the introduction of general anesthesia in the catheterization laboratory is the occurrence of pressure damage and brachial plexus injury when the patient's arms are positioned above the head to facilitate imaging using the lateral camera.[4-6] Care must be taken to pad the table appropriately, and the arms must be moved frequently. Whenever possible, arms should be positioned at the patient's side for part or most of the case, moving them above the head only when absolutely necessary.

Antibiotic coverage (cefazolin, 30 mg/kg, administered in the catheterization laboratory and repeated twice every 6 hours) is provided for interventional procedures involving device or coil placement.[7]

For routine diagnostic catheterizations, the cardiologist will generally prefer that the patient breath spontaneously without supplemental oxygen, to obtain the most realistic assessment of the patient's usual hemodynamic state. However, if a normal pH and partial pressure of carbon dioxide are not maintained, the hemodynamic findings may be meaningless; normal ventilation achieved with mechanical assistance is preferable to respiratory acidosis with a natural airway. For some therapeutic catheterizations, hemodynamic measurements may be limited to a few pertinent questions, and in the perioperative period most children will be sedated, intubated, and mechanically ventilated. Thus, the decision to intubate or refrain from intubating the airway must be individualized, and the decision must be arrived at mutually between the anesthesiologist and the cardiologist.

Routine sedation administered by nonanesthesiologists varies between institutions. At Children's Hospital in Boston, infants weighing <10 kg receive chloral hydrate (75–100 mg/kg), administered orally or rectally, and children weighing between 10 and 20 kg receive "demerol compound" (meperidine, 25 mg; promethazine, 6.25 mg; and chlorpromazine, 6.25 mg/ml) IM up to a maximum of 0.11 ml/kg or 2.0 ml. At Children's Hospital of Philadelphia, the preference is to avoid intramuscular sedation whenever possible; routine precatheterization sedation is achieved, using oral Nembutal (4 mg/kg) and meperidine (3 mg/kg), and this is supplemented as necessary during the procedure, using small doses of intravenous midazolam and morphine. In all cases, local anesthesia (lidocaine, 2%) is given at the site(s) of catheter insertion. Most anesthesiologists prefer to sedate patients with combinations of narcotics and benzodiazepines, titrating doses of morphine (0.05 mg/kg) and midazolam (0.05 mg/kg). If the infant-child is difficult to sedate or requires high doses of medications, ketamine (0.2–0.5 mg/kg) administered by intermittent bolus or by continuous infusion (1 mg/kg/hr) can be used. Ketamine has been demonstrated to have minimal effect on the hemodynamics of patients undergoing cardiac catheterization.[8] Alternatively, in children with good myocardial function who are not dependent on systemic-to-pulmonary shunts or high preload, propofol by intermittent bolus or infusion may be used.[9] Such sedation techniques carry a small but definite risk of airway obstruction.[10,11]

In the postoperative period, sedation alone is rarely used. In these cases, patients usually come to the catheterization laboratory directly from the cardiac ICU and are already sedated, intubated, and often receiving a muscle relaxant. The anesthesiologist's role is mostly to continue adequate sedation, to control ventilation so that arterial gases are kept within acceptable limits, and to monitor supportive therapy. Most of these patients will require positive pressure ventilation in the ICU for some period of time after their procedure.

Preoperatively, most children will tolerate induction of anesthesia with thiopentone, followed by maintenance with inhalational anesthetics and narcotics; we currently use isoflurane with small-to-moderate doses of fentanyl (3–10 mg/kg). Children with depressed myocardial function can be induced with ketamine (1–2 mg/kg). If combined with fentanyl, pancuronium has a minimal effect on heart rate and, in many young children, the relative tachycardia may be an advantage, as the cardiac output is rate dependent. In older children or those already paralyzed, vecuronium as a continuous infusion is frequently used. In children with near terminally depressed myocardial function and depleted catecholamine stores, ketamine may be contraindicated, acting as a direct myocardial depressant.[12–14] In these patients, careful titration with fentanyl and midazolam for induction or, alternatively, etomidate, may be used.[15] Recently, the use of caudal blockade has been proposed for cardiac catheterization. Although initially attractive, this technique does not sedate the child who has to lie still for several hours, and it may alter hemodynamics. Additionally, it does not facilitate insertion of a subclavian or internal jugular vein catheter.

An important part of anesthetic management in the postoperative period is control of PVR and, thus, of pulmonary artery pressure. Hypoventilation with hypercarbia and hypoxemia will increase PVR and worsen (PAH). In an effort to avoid this, children may be moderately hyperventilated aiming at a P_{CO_2} between 30 and 35. However, in the child who has a large left-to-right shunt (for example, an infant who has had repair of tetralogy of Fallot and has large aortopulmonary collateral vessels that need to be coil embolized), hyperventilation will increase the pulmonary-to-systemic flow ratio and may induce hemodynamic instability. Thus, ventilatory management must be adjusted to the individual patient's hemodynamic situation, with one increasing the minute ventilation in situations in which pulmonary blood flow must be augmented and decreasing the minute ventilation when pulmonary blood flow needs to be limited. Other maneuvers that promote a decrease in PVR include adequate sedation with narcotics to protect against stress responses.[16] Recently, the use of inhaled nitric oxide in concentrations of 10 to 80 ppm has been shown to decrease PVR and pulmonary artery pressure in some patients. It may be particularly useful in the postoperative period, as its effectiveness is not diminished by the temporary impairment of endothelial function, which occurs after cardiopulmonary bypass.[17–19] Currently, its use remains investigational.

Most patients who are catheterized in the postoperative period will return directly to the cardiac ICU. The few who are not critically ill may be recovered for a minimum of 30 minutes in a postanesthesia recovery facility, where the patient can be monitored for both emergence from anesthesia and possible adverse events related to the procedure. Hemodynamic status, arterial oxygenation status, respiration, level of consciousness, presence of discomfort, and peripheral pulses are monitored. Parents are encouraged to be present during the recovery phase of the patient. Discomfort, particularly that resulting from the femoral cannulation site and the need for pressure dressing, can be considerable and is treated with opioids; most commonly, we use morphine (0.05 mg/kg), with repeated administration until the patient is comfortable. Nausea and vomiting can be a problem; the straining associated with nausea and vomiting can result in reopening of the femoral cannulation sites. Patients who experience nausea and vomiting will receive either droperidol (75 mg/kg) or ondansetron (150 mg/kg).

GENERAL CONSIDERATIONS IN PERFORMING TRANSCATHETER INTERVENTIONS: THE CARDIOLOGIST'S VIEW

Therapeutic catheterization carries with it certain predictable risks. This chapter is not meant to provide a detailed description of technique for each of the interventions discussed; however, understanding of the tools of the trade (stiff wires, large sheaths, rigid balloons, and implantable devices) and of the basic approach to interventions allows the anesthesiologist to anticipate those portions of the procedure that carry the most risk for the patient and also to recognize when an apparently alarming phenomenon is merely the expected result of the interventionist's actions.

For many procedures, such as dilations and device placement, success of the procedure depends on achieving a stable position of a stiff wire that ends in or passes through the heart. Stretching of the right heart by a stiff wire and/or sheath passing through to the pulmonary artery can result in bradycardia, tricuspid insufficiency, pulmonic insufficiency, or all three. Passage of a wire retrograde into the left ventricle often results in ventricular ectopy, usually in the form of a few premature ventricular contractions or a short run of ventricular ectopy but occasionally in the form of ventricular fibrillation. Passage of a wire, sheath, or catheter through the right heart or retrograde into the left heart will, on occasion, result in complete heart block; this most frequently occurs in transposition of the great arteries (TGA).

The use of large, long sheaths that reach from the neck or groin into the thorax is associated with the risk of embolism of air or thrombus. These events are prevented only by meticulous attention to technique on the part of the catheterizer. The risk of air embolism is significantly reduced by the use of positive pressure ventilation, and that of thromboembolism is reduced by adequate anticoagulation with monitoring of the ACT.[20]

Angioplasty balloons, which are rigid and straight when inflated, are often positioned in curved structures, such as the right ventricular outflow tract or a pulmonary artery. Inflation of the balloon can thus result in stretching of the heart or in rupture of the heart or vessel. In addition, a balloon may traverse several structures, in which case inflation of the balloon may result in inadvertent dilation of a valve, vessel, or septum. Balloon inflation may also result in a transient elimination or severe diminution of cardiac output.

Any implantable device is also a potentially embolic device. Prevention of device embolization is facilitated by keeping the patient immobile. Thus, avoidance of maneuvers such as suctioning of the mouth or endotracheal tube, inflating a blood pressure cuff, engaging in loud conversation in the presence of a sedated (rather than anesthetized) patient, repositioning ECG leads or patient limbs, etc., at the time that an implantable device is being positioned in the heart or vasculature is very helpful to the cardiologist.

SPECIFIC PROCEDURES

Balloon Atrial Septostomy in TGAs

Few innovations in the treatment of children with congenital heart disease have had the impact of balloon atrial septostomy in children with TGA. Before the adoption of this procedure, 1-month survival for infants with TGA was about 50%, and 1-year survival was about 10%. The use of balloon atrial septostomy in the early 1960s allowed infants to survive until they could undergo an atrial level repair (Mustard operation), with a long-term survival of 60 to 90%.[21]

In the current era, the surgical intervention of choice for TGA is the arterial switch operation performed in the neonatal period, making prolonged palliation unnecessary. In addition, the availability of prostaglandin E_1 to maintain patency of the ductus arteriosus often allows adequate mixing without creation of an ASD. Thus, the frequency of balloon atrial septostomy is dramatically reduced. In addition, this procedure is often performed in the ICU under echocardiographic guidance, rather than in the cardiac catheterization laboratory. Nevertheless, centers performing neonatal repair of congenital heart disease will see several newborns each year with TGAs and inadequate mixing due to a restrictive atrial communication. These infants can be critically ill, with arterial Po_2s in the teens and severe metabolic acidosis. Intubation, hyperventilation, and correction of metabolical acidosis must be instituted promptly if the interventionist is to have the opportunity to open the atrial septum.

That balloon atrial septostomy can be performed safely is generally taken for granted; however, the potential risks of the procedure are substantial and may now be increased due to the relative infrequency with which the procedure is performed. The main risk of the procedure is laceration of the heart or great vessels at the time that the balloon is jerked through the septum. Tearing the heart off of the pulmonary veins can occur as a consequence of overinflation of the septostomy balloon,[22] whereas laceration of the inferior vena cava can result from an overly vigorous or poorly controlled tug on the balloon catheter. It is at least theoretically possible to resuscitate the infant from such a catastrophic event if the catheterizer is able to tamponade the laceration with a balloon catheter while the infant is transfused and transported to the operating room.

Creation of an ASD in an Intact Atrial Septum

Periperioperative creation of an ASD may be indicated in a variety of situations. Most often, the patient is one with complex congenital heart disease of the single-ventricle type, with severe mitral hypoplasia or mitral atresia. In this situation, inadequate egress of pulmonary venous blood from the left atrium results in left atrial hypertension and reflex pulmonary artery hypertension; because these patients generally have the ability to shunt from right to left, there will be associated cyanosis, the severity of which is determined by the severity of mitral obstruction. The newborn with critical left heart obstruction and severe mitral stenosis or mitral atresia represents a true interventional emergency; this sort of patient cannot be stabilized unless the atrial septum is opened in the cardiac catheterization laboratory or the operating room. In the older child with less severe mitral obstruction, perioperative relief of left atrial hypertension is desired so that PVR will fall to more normal levels before the child undergoes surgery.

Our approach to this situation is to create an ASD by performing an atrial septal puncture, followed by dilation of the hole with angioplasty balloons. We believe that this approach is more effective and safer than either balloon atrial septostomy after atrial septal puncture or transcatheter blade atrial septostomy. The procedure can be technically quite challenging in the newborn with very small left heart structures. Hyperventilation, correction of metabolic acidosis, and inotropic support are important features of patient management.

Perioperative Dilation or Stenting of Stenotic Pulmonary Arteries

Transcatheter dilation of peripheral pulmonic stenosis was first reported by Lock et al. in 1983[23]; stenting of peripheral pulmonic stenosis was reported in 1988 by Mullins et al.[24] These transcatheter methods of relieving pulmonary artery stenosis are generally reserved for those lesions that are beyond the surgeon's reach or have proven refractory to surgical management. In general, such procedures are performed at times remote from surgical intervention. Transcatheter pulmonary artery dilation is effective only when it results in an intimal and medial tear. These tears are believed to increase the risk of bleeding when the patient is heparinized for cardiopulmonary bypass or if surgery is performed in the same area as the balloon dilation. Transcatheter balloon dilation at or near the surgical site in the immediate postoperative period has been associated with catastrophic pulmonary artery rupture.[25] Nevertheless, these procedures may be performed perioperatively when there is severe hemodynamic instability due to residual branch pulmonary artery stenosis, and it is believed that surgical intervention involves excessive risk or is unlikely to be effective. In such instances, the patient is likely to have a very low cardiac output, and either right ventricular hypertension or severe right ventricular dysfunction, or both. Anesthetic management is focused on maneuvers that will lower PVR and minimize oxygen consumption.

Preoperative Closure of Unwanted Vascular Communications

Unwanted vascular communications in children with congenital heart disease can include patent ductus arteriosus, aortopulmonary collaterals, veno-venous collaterals, left superior venae cavae, surgically created aortopulmonary shunts, and pulmonary arteriovenous malformations; any of these may be amenable to transcatheter occlusion.[26,27] Elimination of these communications before surgery may be desirable for one or more of the following reasons: to allow the surgeon to avoid an extensive dissection into the left or right chest; to reduce the amount of blood returning to the heart while the patient is on cardiopulmonary bypass and allow for more even cooling of the upper body on cardiopulmonary bypass; or to avoid having to perform both a medial sternotomy and a lateral thoracotomy. Elimination of these communications postoperatively may be necessary for one or more of the following reasons: the vascular communication allows enough left-to-right shunting to result in congestive heart failure; the vascular communication results in elevated pulmonary artery pressure, which is not tolerated in a particular hemodynamic setting (e.g., in a patient who has had a Fontan operation); or the vascular communication allows enough right-to-left shunting to result in intolerable cyanosis.

In general, such vascular communications are closed with coils. Accurate imaging and measurement of the vessel to be closed are crucial in helping one to choose a coil of appropriate size; a coil that is too large will fail to curl up when placed in the vessel, and thus will not be occlusive, whereas one that is too small is likely to result in an embolism.

At times, an aortopulmonary connection will be embolized in the catheterization laboratory immediately before a patient is taken to surgery; this is done when it is anticipated that the patient will tolerate elimination of that vessel only for a limited time, and then only if under general anesthesia; it is done so that oxygen consumption is minimized, and ventilation and oxygenation are maximized.

Device Closure of Postoperative Residual ASDs or Baffle Leaks

The first successful transcatheter closure of an ASD in a patient was reported by King et al. in 1976.[28] Subsequently, a variety of double-umbrella devices for closure of intracardiac defects has been designed and successfully used,[29–31] although none is yet available, except under very restrictive investigational protocols. Where available, such devices may be used for closure of postoperative residual ASDs or atrial baffle leaks that result in hemodynamic compromise in the immediate postoperative period. The main advantage of such an approach over surgery is the avoidance of a second period of cardiopulmonary bypass. Hundreds of transcatheter procedures for closure of ASDs have been performed, and the procedure is safe and effective in experienced hands. Potential risks of the procedure include air and/or device embolization, as well as peripheral vascular injury; adequate sedation or general anesthesia with positive pressure ventilation reduces these risks, and ASD closure is generally associated with few hemodynamic problems.[11] General anesthesia is not routine, unless transesophageal echocardiography is necessary to assist in positioning the device or with patients who have limited hemodynamic reserve. Hypotension and rhythm disturbances are uncommon, and transfusion is rarely required. Sedation, along with local anesthesia to the groin, is usually satisfactory; however, patients must be still during device placement and, occasionally, administration of a bolus of ketamine (1 to 2 mg/kg) or propofol is necessary at this time.

Perioperative Closure of VSDs

Surgical closure of most types of VSDs is accomplished with a vanishingly small risk of reoperation or death; however, this is not the case for some muscular VSDs, particularly those associated with complex congenital heart lesions. For this reason, these defects are sometimes closed, using a transcatheter technique, before or after surgical repair of other congenital heart lesions. Postoperative transcatheter closure of hemodynamically significant residual VSDs, particularly those in the anterior muscular septum or at a patch margin, is also occasionally undertaken.[32] Transesophageal echocardiography is frequently used to determine the position of the device arms and to evaluate residual shunting and atrioventricular valve function.

Transcatheter VSD device closures can be prolonged procedures, associated with significant hemodynamic instability and blood loss. Transfusion has been required in more than half of the patients undergoing these procedures at Children's Hospital in Boston, with most of those requiring transfusion weighing less than 10 kg. Hypotension (defined as more than 20% fall in systolic blood pressure from baseline) occurred in almost half of the patients as well. Significant arrhythmias associated with hypotension and desaturation occurred in about 30% of the patients. These included ventricular arrhythmias requiring treatment with lidocaine, as well as junctional bradycardia or complete heart block requiring treatment with transvenous pacing and/or isoproterenol.[33]

Initially patients undergoing these procedures were managed with sedation; however, as our experience with these procedures has increased, general anesthesia has replaced sedation. Intensive care management is frequently required after transcatheter VSD closure.

TRANSCATHETER ABLATION

Transcatheter ablation of accessory pathways or automatic foci, using RF energy, is an effective method of treating many reentrant and automatic dysrhythmias. RF energy is a low-power, high-frequency alternating current that causes controlled injury by creating heat at the tip of the catheter. In contrast to direct current, which can cause intense retrosternal pain, RF ablation is virtually painless. Although most often used in structurally normal hearts as an alternative to surgery, RF ablation is also used pre- and postoperatively to abolish dysrhythmias that occur in children with structural congenital heart disease.[34,35] In a recent multicenter study from the Pediatric Electrophysiology Society, approximately 15% of children undergoing RF ablation procedures had structural congenital heart defects. RF catheter ablation was effective and safe in these patients.[36]

There is an extensive body of literature about anesthetic agents and their cardiovascular effects, but there is little about the effect of these agents on the normal conduction system. Most studies have been performed in adults, using surface electrocardiography, and have been limited to the proarrhythmic properties of anesthetic agents, in combination with endogenous and exogenous catecholamines.[37] Studies of intravenous agents showed that fentanyl, alfentanil, and midazolam had no effect on the accessory pathway refractory period in patients with Wolff-Parkinson-White syndrome, whereas droperidol increased the refractory period.[38] A similar study performed during surgical ablation of accessory pathways in patients with Wolff-Parkinson-White syndrome studied the effects of volatile anesthetic agents and sufentanil.[39] Sufentanil (20 mg/kg), combined with lorazepam (0.06 mg/kg), had no clinically important effect on the accessory pathway. A study of volatile agents demonstrated that enflurane (strongest effect), then isoflurane, and halothane (least effect) increased refractoriness within the accessory and normal atrioventricular pathways.[40] A recent study, comparing the effects of isoflurane and propofol with those of baseline anesthesia (alfentanil-N_2O-pancuronium) in 20 children with supraventricular tachycardia, demonstrated no effect on electrophysiological measurements.[41]

Anesthetic management of patients with structural heart defects who are undergoing RF ablation depends on their cardiac pathophysiology. After the procedure, these patients are more likely to require an overnight stay in the cardiac ICU than are patients with structurally normal hearts; the latter are generally extubated in the cardiac catheterization laboratory and recover in a PACU.

CONCLUSION

The introduction of interventional techniques has revolutionized the treatment of congenital heart defects. Collaboration between cardiac surgeons, cardiac interventionists, and cardiac anesthesiologists ideally begins before the performance of any intervention and continues until the patient is stable with respect to airway and hemodynamic issues. This sort of approach results in a therapeutic strategy that is greater than the sum of its parts and maximizes the potential for a good outcome in children with complex or critical heart disease.

References

1. Bing RJ, Vandam L, Gray FD Jr: Physiological studies in congenital heart disease. I. Procedures. Bull Johns Hopkins Hosp 80:107–120, 1947
2. Dotter CT, Judkins MP: Transluminal treatment of arteriosclerotic obstruction. Description of a new technique and a preliminary report of its application. Circulation 30:654–679, 1964
3. Rashkind WJ, Miller WW: Creation of an atrial septal defect without thoracotomy: Palliative approach to complete transposition of the great arteries. JAMA 196:991–992, 1966
4. Bridges ND, Lock JE, Castaneda AR: Baffle fenestration with subsequent transcatheter closure: Modification of the Fontan operation for patients at increased risk. Circulation 82:1681–1689, 1990
5. Bridges ND, Perry SB, Keane JF et al: Preoperative transcatheter closure of congenital muscular ventricular septal defects. N Engl J Med 324:1312–1317, 1991
6. Hickey PR, Wessel DL, Streitz SL, Fox ML, Kern FH, Bridges ND, Hansen DD: Transcatheter closure of atrial septal defects: Hemodynamic complications and anesthetic management. Anesth Analg 74:44–50, 1992
7. Dajani AS, Bisno AL, Chung KJ et al: Prevention of bacterial endocarditis: Recommendations by the American Heart Association. JAMA 264:2919–2922, 1990
8. Morray JP, Lynn AM, Stamm SJ, Herndon PS, Kawabori I, Stevenson JG: Hemodynamic effects of ketamine in children with congenital heart disease. Anesth Analg 63:895–899, 1984
9. Smith I, White PF, Nathanson M, Gouldson R: Propofol: An update on its clinical use. Anesthesiology 81:1005–1043, 1994
10. Hickey PR, Wessel DL, Streitz SL et al: Transcatheter closure of atrial septal defects: Hemodynamic complications and anesthetic management. Anesth Analg 74:44–50, 1992
11. Malviya S, Burrows FA, Johnston AE, Benson LN: Anaesthetic experience with paediatric interventional cardiology. Can J Anaesth 36:320–324, 1989
12. Miletich DJ, Ivankovic AD, Labrecht RF, Zahed B, Ilahi AA: The effect of ketamine on catecholamine metabolism in the isolated perfused rat heart. Anesthesiology 39:271–277, 1973
13. Nedergaard OA: Cocaine-like effect of ketamine on vascular adrenergic neurones. Eur J Pharmacol 23:153–161, 1973
14. Urthaler F, Walker AA, James TN: Comparison of the inotropic action of morphine and ketamine. J Thorac Cardiovasc Surg 72:142–149, 1976
15. Schechter WS, Kim C, Martinez M, Gleason BF, Lind DP, Burrows FA: Anaesthetic induction in a child with end-stage cardiomyopathy. Can J Anaesth 42:404–408, 1995

16. Hickey PR, Hansen DD, Wessel DL, Lang P, Jonas RA, Elixson EM: Blunting of stress responses in the pulmonary circulation of infants by fentanyl. Anesth Analg 64:1137–1142, 1985

17. Frostell CG, Fratacci MD, Win JC, Jones R, Zapol WM: Inhaled NO: A selective pulmonary vasodilator reversing hypoxic pulmonary vasoconstriction. Circulation 83:2038–2047, 1991

18. Roberts JD, Polaner DM, Lang P, Zapol WM: Inhaled nitric oxide in PPHN. Lancel 240:818–819, 1992

19. Roberts JD, Lang P, Bigatello LM, Vlahakas GJ, Zapol WM: Inhaled nitric oxide in congenital heart disease. Circulation 87:447–453, 1993

20. Grady RM, Eisenberg PR, Bridges ND: Rational approach to use of heparin during cardiac catheterization in children. J Am Coll Cardiol 25:725–729, 1995

21. Paul MH, Wernovsky G: Transposition of the great arteries. In Emmanouilides, Allen, Reimenschneider, and Gutgesell (eds): Moss and Adams' Heart Disease in Infants, Children and Adolescents, including the fetus and Young Adult, 5th ed., p. 1154. Baltimore, Williams & Wilkins, 1995

22. Sondheimer HM, Kavey REW, Blackman MS: Fatal overdistension of an atrioseptostomy catheter. Pediatr Cardiol 2:255, 1982

23. Lock JE, Castaneda-Zuniga WR, Fuhrman BP, Bass JL: Balloon dilation angioplasty of hypoplastic and stenotic pulmonary arteries. Circulation 67:962–967, 1983

24. O'Laughlin MP, Perry SB, Lock JE, Mullins CE: Use of endovascular stents in congenital heart disease. Circulation 83:1923–1939, 1991

25. Rothman A, Perry SB, Keane JF, Lock JE: Early results and follow-up of balloon angioplasty for branch pulmonary artery stenosis. J Am Coll Cardiol 15:1109–1117, 1990

26. Fuhrman BP, Bass JL, Castaneda-Zuniga W, Amplatz K, Lock JE: Coil embolization of congenital thoracic vascular anomalies in infants and children. Circulation 70:285–289, 1984

27. Perry SB, Radtke W, Fellows KE, Keane JF, Lock JE: Coil embolization to occlude aortopulmonary collateral vessels and shunts in patients with congenital heart disease. J Am Coll Cardiol 13:100–108, 1989

28. King TD, Thompson SL, Steiner CS, Mills NL: Secundum atrial septal defect: Nonoperative closure during cardiac catheterization. JAMA 235:2506–2509, 1976

29. Rashkind WJ: Transcatheter treatment of congenital heart disease. Circulation 67:711–716, 1983

30. Rome JJ, Keane JF, Perry SB, Spevak PJ, Lock JE: Double-umbrella closure of atrial defects: Initial clinical applications. Circulation 82:751–758, 1990

31. Rao PS, Wilson AD, Chopra PS: Transcatheter closure of atrial septral defect by "buttoned" devices. Am J Cardiol 69:1056–1061, 1992

32. Lock JE, Block PB, McKay RG, Baim DS, Keane JF: Transcatheter closure of ventricular septal defects. Circulation 78:361–368, 1988

33. Laussen PC, Hansen DD, Perry SB et al: Transcatheter closure of ventricular septal defects: Hemodynamic instability and anesthetic management. Anesth Analg 80:1076–1082, 1995

34. Van Hare GF, Lesh MD, Stanger P: Radiofrequency catheter ablation of supraventricular arrhythmias in patients with congenital heart disease: Results and technical considerations. J Am Coll Cardiol 22:883–890, 1993

35. Levine JC, Walsh EP, Saul JP: Radiofrequency ablation of accessory pathways associated with congenital heart disease including heterotaxy syndrome. Am J Cardiol 72:689–693, 1993

36. Kugler JD, Danford DA, Deal BJ et al: Radiofrequency catheter ablation for tachyarrhythmias in children and adolescents. N Engl J Med 330: 1481–1487, 1949
37. Atlee JL III, Bosnjak ZK: Mechanism for cardiac dysrhythmias during anesthesia.
38. Gomez-Arnau J, Marquez-Montes J, Avello F: Fentanyl and droperidol effects on the refractoriness of the accessory pathway in the Wolff-Parkinson-White syndrome. Anesthesiology 58:307–313, 1983
39. Sharpe MD, Dobkowski WB, Murkin JM, Klein G, Guiraudon G, Yee R: Alfentanil-midazolam anaesthesia has no electrophysiological effects upon the normal conduction system or accessory pathways in patients with Wolff-Parkinson-White syndrome. Can J Anaesth 39:816–821, 1992
40. Sharpe MD, Dobkowski WB, Murkin JM, Klein G, Guiraudon G, Yee R: The electrophysiological effects of volatile anesthetics and sufentanil on the normal atrioventricular conduction system and accessory pathways in Wolff-Parkinson-White syndrome. Anesthesiology 80:63–70, 1994
41. Lavoie J, Walsh EP, Burrows FA, Laussen PC, Lulu JA, Hansen DD: Effects of propofol or isoflurane anesthesia on cardiac conduction in children undergoing radiofrequency catheter ablation for tachydysrhythmias. Anesthesiology 82:884–887, 1995

Victor C. Baum

Noncardiac Surgery for the Adult Patient with Congenital Heart Disease

8

Over the past four decades the phenomenal advances made in the surgical and perioperative care of children born with congenital heart disease have enabled the vast majority of these children to grow into adulthood. As an example, the survival data from a large group of children referred to a single institution from 1952 to 1963 with 26- to 37-year follow-up is shown in Figure 8–1 (from ref. 1). Currently, more than 500,000 adults in the United States are estimated to be with congenital heart disease, and every year more than 20,000 intracardiac operations for congenital heart disease are done in the United States.[2–5] More than 85% of the 25,000 children born in the United States each year with congenital heart disease can be expected to reach adulthood.

As these patients reach adulthood, and eventually, old age, they will be seen by anesthesiologists in the operating room not only for cardiac operations but also for the entire spectrum of surgical procedures (Fig. 8–2). In anesthetizing these patients, one must be cognizant not only of the physiological implications of the underlying cardiac defect(s), which may change with time, but also of the cardiac and noncardiac residua and sequelae of prior surgery, as well as the acquired cardiac and noncardiac diseases that accrue with normal aging. Perioperative cardiac care has occurred on a dynamic, improving continuum. The long-term results of surgery have been affected by a variety of factors, such as improved intraoperative myocardial protection

Perioperative Management of the Patient with Congenital Heart Disease, edited by William J. Greeley. Williams & Wilkins, Baltimore © 1996.

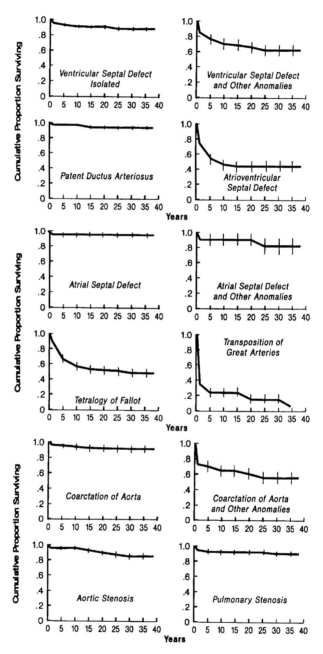

FIGURE 8–1. Long-term survival in the era of cardiac surgery for a variety of congenital cardiac defects referred to a single institution. *(Adapted with permission from The American Journal of Cardiology. Moller JH, Anderson RC. Am J Cardiol, 70:661–667, 1992)*

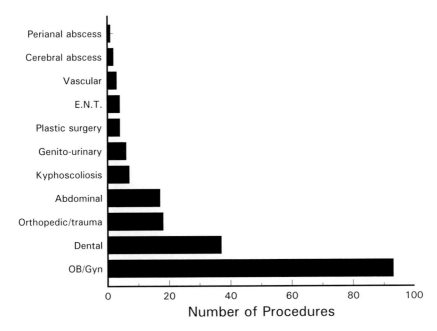

FIGURE 8–2. The distribution of noncardiac surgical procedures in a group of adolescent patients with congenital heart disease. As this group ages, the distribution of surgical procedures would be expected to shift somewhat. E.N.T., ear, nose, and throat. *(Reprinted with permission from the American College of Cardiology (Journal of the American College of Cardiology, 1991; 18:324))*

and surgery at younger ages, so all natural history data must be interpreted in an appropriate historical light.

Although most adult patients with congenital heart disease will have had some type of surgical intervention, of which, many have been labeled as "corrective," there are, in fact, very few lesions that, on an absolute population-wide basis, are considered to be amenable to absolute cure.[6,7] Cure in this context requires the achievement and maintenance of normal cardiac function and life expectancy, and further medical or surgical management of the congenital cardiac lesion is not required. The very few examples of cure are uncomplicated closure of a nonpulmonary hypertensive patent ductus arteriosus and closure of an uncomplicated secundum atrial septal defect.

Before undertaking the anesthetic care of adults with congenital heart disease, clearly an appreciation of the anatomy and physiology of congenital cardiac lesions is required. Pediatric cardiac anesthesia is the foundation on which care of the adult with congenital heart disease is built, and one's understanding of basic pediatric cardiac anesthesia must be firmly grounded. Several widely available texts include complete descriptions of these lesions and their surgical palliation and repair.[8-10] Similarly, pediatric cardiac anesthesia is the topic of chapters in the larger anesthesia texts, as well as in several subspecialty texts.[11,12] A discussion of the natural history of the large number of congenital heart defects and their variants and subtypes, as well as the very unnatural history of the surgically altered heart, is, unfortunately, beyond the scope of this chapter, and the reader is directed to a number of sources for this information.[13-17] Similarly, the effects of congenital heart disease and pregnancy and delivery, another common source of interaction of the anesthesiology service with adults with congenital heart disease, is also not discussed here, and interested readers are referred to several recent discussions.[18-23]

The remainder of this chapter, then, will consider primarily the noncardiac manifestations of congenital heart disease in the adult, which are perhaps less well appreciated by anesthesiologists. In addition, a section is devoted to Eisenmenger physiology, often found in adult patients referred for anesthetic evaluation, and a final section will discuss general perioperative considerations associated with adults with congenital heart disease.

NONCARDIAC ORGAN SYSTEM MANIFESTATIONS

Pulmonary Interactions

Potential pulmonary manifestations of longstanding congenital heart disease are summarized in Table 8–1. Cardiac defects that cause increased pulmonary blood flow as the result of left-to-right shunting can result in decreased pulmonary compliance,[24] which, in turn, increases the work of breathing. Small bronchioles may be partially obstructed, resulting in what has been called in the past "cardiac

TABLE 8–1. POTENTIAL RESPIRATORY MANIFESTATIONS

Decreased pulmonary compliance with left-to-right shunts
Small bronchiolar collapse with airway obstruction
Blunted response to hypoxemia with cyanotic disease
Underestimation of arterial P_{CO_2} by capnometry with cyanotic disease
Compression of bronchi by large hypertensive pulmonary arteries
Diaphragmatic paresis-paralysis from prior thoracic surgery
Recurrent laryngeal nerve injury from prior surgery or impaction by pulmonary artery
Scoliosis
Upper lobe pulmonary artery thrombosis with Eisenmenger physiology
Hemoptysis in end-stage Eisenmenger physiology

asthma." Interestingly, there has not been significant investigation into the ventilatory response to hypercarbia in patients with chronic cyanosis, although there has been some investigation of normal subjects hypoxemic at high altitude.[25] Patients with chronic cyanosis tend to have increased ventilation with normal $Paco_2$.[26] Although chronically cyanosed patients have a normal ventilatory response to hypercarbia, they manifest a blunted response to hypoxemia, as might be expected,[27,28] which resolves with normoxemia following surgical correction.[29] End-tidal Pco_2 accurately represents $Paco_2$ in acyanotic patients with normal or increased pulmonary blood flow; however, capnometry systematically underestimates $Paco_2$ in cyanotic patients with decreased, normal, or increased pulmonary blood flow.[30]

Left-to-right shunts resulting in large, hypertensive pulmonary arteries can cause chronic compression of bronchi in children, resulting in recurrent or chronic atelectasis, pneumonia, or focal emphysema,[31] although this is much less common in adults. Several sites are at risk for compression. The left pulmonary artery can compress the left mainstem and upper lobe bronchi, and the right middle lobe bronchus can be compressed by a large hypertensive right lower lobe pulmonary artery. Chronic atelectasis-pneumonia of the right lower lobe from bronchial compression is the so-called right middle lobe syndrome. Similarly, the left mainstem and upper lobe bronchi can be compressed between the left upper lobe pulmonary artery and a large left atrium.

In addition to the above, an enlarged hypertensive main pulmonary artery can compress the recurrent laryngeal nerve. Hemoptysis and upper lobe thrombosis are complications of Eisenmenger physiology with severe pulmonary arterial hypertension. Patients who have had prior thoracic surgery may have diaphragmatic paresis or paralysis from phrenic nerve injury.

Congenital cardiac defects often exist as but one component of a dysmorphic syndrome which may also have pulmonary manifestations. Aboussouan et al., for example, surveyed a group of adult patients with Down syndrome both with and without cardiac disease. They found decreased tracheal diameters in these adult patients (previously described in pediatric patients with Down syndrome) that were unrelated to body habitus or the presence of cardiac disease.[32]

Scoliosis not uncommonly develops in patients with congenital heart disease, particularly cyanotic disease, with incidence reported to be as high as 19%,[33] and many of these patients will have surgical repair of their back deformity. Scoliosis typically develops during adolescence, even when the cyanosis had been relieved by surgery years before. The degree of scoliosis is only rarely severe enough to significantly impair pulmonary function, however.

The development of pulmonary arteriovenous fistulae was a problem with the original Glenn cavopulmonary anastomosis (end-to-end superior vena cava to right pulmonary artery). These fistulae could, on occasion, be quite large and numerous and in themselves be a cause of cyanosis. Although it seems that current modifications of the Glenn shunt (the bidirectional Glenn) and the Fontan procedure result in a significantly decreased incidence of fistulae. However, they can still occur,[34] particularly when looked for diligently.[35] Their cause is unknown. It has been hypothesized that it may be related to the exclusion of hepatic venous blood from pulmonary circulation.

Fluid retention with pleural effusion is common after the Fontan operation in children. One series reported persistent fluid accumulations in 28% of adult patients who have had a Fontan procedure.[36]

Hematological Interactions

Chronic cardiac disease may adversely affect the hematological system. These are listed in Table 8–2. Although most of the interactions are related to chronic hypoxemia, there are also some effects in patients with acyanotic disease. In patients with chronic hypoxemia the oxygen-hemoglobin dissociation curve is normal or slightly right shifted,[37] and there is a poor relationship between oxygen saturation, 2,3-diphosphoglycerate (DPG) levels, and red cell mass.[38] Most patients with cyanotic congenital heart disease establish an equilibrium that is adequate for oxygen delivery, have a stable hematocrit, and are iron replete. Some patients, however, do not establish an equilibrium, have excessive hematocrit levels, and may be iron deficient. As an aside, patients with cyanotic heart disease are typically *erythrocytotic*, rather than *polycythemic*, as they have an increase only in red cell number (erythrocytosis) and not in all blood elements (polycythemia).

The major sequelae associated with high hematocrit are related to the development of hyperviscosity. If the patient is iron replete, hyperviscosity is rarely symptomatic if the hematocrit is less than 65%.

TABLE 8–2. HEMATOLOGICAL INTERACTIONS

Erythrocytosis with hyperviscosity
Artifactually elevated manually measured hematocrit with erythrocytosis
Bleeding dyscrasias due to blood or tissue factors
Artifactual thrombocytopenia
Artifactual elevations in PT and PTTs
Abnormal von Willebrand factor
Gallstone formation

Symptoms of hyperviscosity include headache; faintness; dizziness; lightheadedness; blurred vision or diplopia; fatigue; myalgias; muscle weakness; paresthesias of fingers, toes, or lips; and depressed mentation or a feeling of dissociation.

Thrombosis would seem to be a concern in patients with excessive erythrocytosis, and cerebral venous thrombosis is associated with erythrocytosis and hyperviscosity in children under 4 years of age. Adults with cyanotic disease, however, are not at risk for cerebral venous or arterial thrombosis, regardless of the level of hematocrit (see Neurological Function, below).[39] Thrombosis may occur, however, in upper lobe pulmonary arteries in patients who also have pulmonary vascular disease, such as would be found with Eisenmenger physiology with right-to-left shunting.

If hyperviscosity symptoms develop, and are clearly related to an elevated hematocrit not due to volume contraction from dehydration, for example, isovolumic phlebotomy is recommended for temporary relief. Phlebotomy is recommended not for a given hematocrit but rather to be based on the development of symptoms referable to hyperviscosity. Reductions in hematocrit have been shown to result in transient improvement in systemic blood flow, stroke volume, and oxygen transport.[39-41] Isovolumic phlebotomy is performed by the removal of 500 ml of blood with replacement by crystalloid or colloid. Symptoms of hyperviscosity generally resolve within 24 hours. It is unusual for a patient to require the removal of more than one unit of blood.

Iron deficiency is a potentiating factor in the development of hyperviscosity. Iron-deficient red cells are less deformable than are iron replete red cells and, thus, for any level of hematocrit blood viscosity will be higher.[42-44] Iron deficiency may be related to relatively deficient intake in cyanotic children but in the adult is typically related to excessive inappropriate phlebotomies. It is reflected in microcytic hypochromic red blood cells despite erythrocytosis. Treatment with oral iron is occasionally required but should be undertaken with extreme caution and diligence as major increases in hematocrit can occur.

Dehydration in an otherwise asymptomatic erythrocytotic patient can result in a rapid increase in the hematocrit level and the development of hyperviscosity symptoms. The treatment of erythrocytosis in the setting is, of course, repletion of intravascular volume. Excessive preoperative fasting needs to be avoided in patients with significantly elevated hematocrit levels. This should not be a problem, with newer recommendations allowing briefer periods of preoperative fasting.

In the presence of erythrocytosis, the hematocrit measured by a microhematocrit tube may be falsely high due to plasma trapping,[45] and hematocrit should be measured by automated machines. Clinical chemistry laboratories may require more blood than usual due to the diminished volume of plasma or serum present in each volume of erythrocytotic blood, as compared to that in normal blood.

Excessive surgical bleeding is a common finding in erythrocytotic cyanotic patients and a variety of hemostatic abnormalities have been described.[46] Although significant bleeding can occur with major trauma or surgery at lesser degrees of erythrocytosis, major bleeding diatheses are usually mild or absent until the hematocrit increases to greater than 65%. Despite investigation, the exact mechanisms of hemostatic defects have not yet been fully defined.

Platelet counts in erythrocytotic patients are generally in the normal range but are occasionally reported to be low. Bleeding is not typically due to thrombocytopenia. When corrected for the smaller amount of plasma in each volume of blood, the actual platelet count (per milliliter of plasma) is typically closer to normal (Fig. 8–3). This situation is analogous to the pseudohyponatremia reported with hyperlipidemia. Abnormalities of platelet function have, however, been reported on occasion.[47–50] Patients with synthetic vascular anastomoses, for example, modified Blalock-Taussig anastomoses constructed from Goretex, are sometimes maintained on a platelet inhibitor (aspirin), which may also increase the degree of intraoperative bleeding.

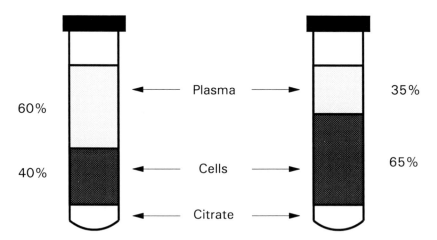

FIGURE 8–3. Illustration of the effect of a fixed amount of citrate anticoagulant in tubes of blood with normal and increased hematocrit. The fixed anticoagulant volume with decreased plasma volume in the erythrocytotic blood results in artifactual elevation of PTs and PTTs. Similarly, although the concentrations of platelets is identical in both samples of *plasma*, the platelet count *per ml of whole blood* (which is reported by the laboratory) will be lower in erythrocytotic blood. *(Reproduced with permission from Baum VC. J Cardiothorac Vasc Anesth, in press, 1996)*

A variety of abnormalities of both the intrinsic and extrinsic clotting cascades have been described in patients with chronic cyanosis.[50–54] The fibrinolytic system is normal.[55] On occasion, deficiencies of the largest von Willebrand multimers have been described in both cyanotic and acyanotic patients,[56] which have normalized after corrective surgery.[57]

Preoperative measurements of prothrombin and partial thromboplastin times (PT and PTT) are frequently obtained preoperatively. However, in the face of significant erythrocytosis the results of these tests, if done in the routine manner, will be inaccurate. Tubes for the determination of PT and PTT contain a fixed amount of citrate as an anticoagulant. This volume presupposes a normal hematocrit level but will be excessive for the amount of plasma in erythrocytotic blood, as each milliliter of blood contains relatively more red cells and, therefore, less plasma (shown in Fig. 8–3). This problem is, however, easily remedied. If the laboratory technicians are informed of the patient's hematocrit, they can prepare a tube in advance with an amount of anticoagulant appropriate for the degree of the patient's erythrocytosis. This correction should be done whenever hematocrit levels are greater than 55%. Correcting to an idealized hematocrit of 45% (plasma volume of 55%), the following formula can be used to calculate the correct amount of citrate to add to the tube:

$$1 \text{ ml of Citrate} = (0.1 \times \text{Blood Volume Collected}) \times \frac{(100 - \text{Patient's Hematocrit})}{55}$$

In the occasional, markedly erythrocytotic patient, isovolumic phlebotomy may be indicated to reduce the hematocrit level to improve perioperative hemostasis.[39] A 500-ml isovolumic phlebotomy is performed every day until a hematocrit level of just under 65% is obtained. With appropriate coordination within the hospital, the phlebotomized blood can be banked for autologous perioperative transfusion if needed.

In addition to the intrinsic hemostatic defects detailed above, there are additional factors present that may result in excessive perioperative blood loss; these include the increased tissue vascularity seen in cyanotic patients, elevated systemic venous pressure due to the underlying cardiac process, and the development of aorta-to-pulmonary and transpleural collateral vessels, which serve to increase pulmonary blood flow in patients with inadequate pulmonary blood flow. In addition, most of these patients will have had prior palliative or corrective thoracic procedures, also increasing the risk of excessive bleeding with or without unintended entry by the surgeon into large vessels or cardiac chambers during subsequent thoracic procedures.

Because of the abnormal hemoglobin turnover, adults with cyanotic heart disease have an increased incidence of calcium bilirubinate gallstone formation, which may express itself as acute cholecystitis. Biliary colic may develop years after cardiac surgery and resolution of the cyanosis.

Renal Function

Patients with chronic cyanosis will develop histological changes in the renal glomeruli, marked by hypercellular glomeruli with basement membrane thickening, focal interstitial fibrosis, tubular atrophy, and hyalinization of both afferent and efferent arterioles.[58] High plasma uric acid levels in adults with cyanotic disease are due to low fractional uric acid excretion, rather than to urate overproduction, as might have been expected in the face of high hematocrits.[59] Enhanced uric acid reabsorption probably is the result of both renal hypoperfusion and a high filtration fraction. Thus, hyperuricemia serves as a marker of abnormal intrarenal hemodynamics.

Although serum uric acid levels are elevated, urate nephropathy and urate stones are rare.[60] Arthralgias are common in patients with chronic cyanosis and are probably related to hypertrophic osteoarthropathy, as true gouty arthritis is not common and less so than would be expected from the levels of plasma uric acid that are seen.[59]

Neurological Function

Patients with congenital heart disease may present with a variety of problems of the central or peripheral nervous systems referable to their cardiac disease (Table 8–3). Two major complications that may occur in adult patients with defects that allow for continuous or potential right-to-left shunting are brain abscess and "paradoxical" cerebral embolization. Adult patients with right-to-left shunting remain liable to develop brain abscesses, which may require operative drainage. A brain abscess in childhood that heals may have a seizure dis-

TABLE 8–3. POTENTIAL NEUROLOGICAL PROBLEMS

Brain abscess: New or sequelae from old
Paradoxical emboli
Hemorrhage from circle of Willis aneurysm with coarctation
Subclavian steal with Blalock-Taussig anastomosis
Injury to recurrent laryngeal nerve, phrenic nerve, or sympathetic chain from
   prior thoracic operations

order as a sequela in adulthood.[61] Emboli from lower extremity thrombosis developing in the poorly mobile postoperative adult patient serve as a source of paradoxical emboli to the brain. Another potential source of emboli is from the introduction of air or particles into venous catheters.

Young children under the age of 4 years with right-to-left shunting lesions are at risk to develop cerebral thromboses. Fortunately, but for unclear reasons, older patients are not at such risk. Following 112 adult patients with cyanotic congenital heart disease, Perloff and his colleagues could find no instances of cerebral thrombosis, independent of the degree of erythrocytosis or the presence of hyperviscosity symptoms.[62] Thus, phlebotomy is not indicated to reduce the risk of cerebral thrombosis in adult patients, as such risk does not exist, and there are very real risks to repeated unnecessary phlebotomy.

An additional potential complication is a cerebral hemorrhage at a circle of Willis aneurysm in patients with coarctation of the aorta.[63] Most patients with coarctation who die of a cerebral hemorrhage are in their 2nd or 3rd decade. A cerebral hemorrhage can occur years after a successful correction of the coarctation and in the absence of hypertension.

A rare complication after the creation of a Blalock-Taussig anastomosis is the presence of a subclavian steal.[64] The classic Blalock-Taussig anastomosis may create an anatomical and physiological parallel of subclavian steal secondary to atherosclerotic disease of the proximal subclavian artery. Symptomatic steal may develop decades after the creation of the anastomosis, depending on the development of collateral vessels.

A hypertensive distended pulmonary artery can impact on the recurrent laryngeal nerve, as detailed in the section on pulmonary interactions. In addition, prior intrathoracic procedures, particularly at the apices of the thorax, such as the creation of a Blalock-Taussig anastomosis, closure of a patent ductus arteriosus, or repair of a coarctation of the aorta, may result in injury to the recurrent laryngeal nerve with subsequent hoarseness, to the phrenic nerve with ipsilateral diaphragmatic paresis or palsy, or to the sympathetic chain with the development of ipsilateral Horner's syndrome. Obviously, these should be looked for on the preoperative physical examination and documented on the preoperative note.

EISENMENGER PHYSIOLOGY

One of the most feared and irreparable complications of congenital heart disease is the development of pulmonary vascular disease with abnormally elevated pulmonary vascular resistance. Eisenmenger

originally described a very specific type of nonrestrictive ventriculoseptal defect, and the term Eisenmenger syndrome was used to describe patients with nonrestrictive ventriculoseptal defect, pulmonary
vascular disease, and reversed shunt. Subsequently, the use of Eisenmenger syndrome or Eisenmenger physiology has been used somewhat more generically to describe patients with pulmonary vascular
disease, regardless of the level of shunt. Eisenmenger physiology is
compatible with survival into adulthood.[65]

This elevation in pulmonary vascular resistance is the hemodynamic manifestation of physiological and anatomical changes in the
pulmonary arterial vasculature.[66,67] During gestation, the pulmonary
arteries become muscularized centrifugally, such that by term, arteries
as small as 180 μm have muscularized media. During the first or second month of life, this muscularization regresses in the normal neonate, accounting for the decrease in pulmonary vascular resistance
manifested over this period. Lesions that are manifested by increases
in the shear force of blood in the pulmonary arteries will cause delayed regression of this musculature. Early during the course, these
changes are reversible, either acutely by pharmacological means or
permanently through surgical correction. With time, specific anatomical changes take place, and the elevated pulmonary vascular resistance is not only irreversible but also may be progressive, despite
surgical correction. Surgical correction in the face of significantly elevated, irreversible pulmonary hypertension may be fatal with the development of acute right-sided failure.

The time course for the development of pulmonary vascular disease is dependent on shear force. As such, it is dependent on flow,
force, and time. Thus lesions such as a large ventriculoseptal defect
or truncus arteriosus with high-flow and high-pressure shunts may
develop irreversible changes in the first year or few years of life,
whereas a patient with a large atrial septal defect may not develop
pulmonary hypertension until latter middle age.

The presence of pulmonary hypertension and elevated pulmonary vascular resistance can be documented by cardiac catheterization
or echocardiography-Doppler interrogation of the heart and can be
inferred from the physical examination (single or narrowly split second heart sound with a loud pulmonic component, Graham-Steel
murmur of pulmonary insufficiency, pulmonic ejection sound
("click")). Suggestive findings may also be present on the electrocardiogram (right ventricular and possibly right atrial hypertrophy) and
on the chest radiograph (prominent main pulmonary artery and
branches with "pruning," or a rapid decrement in size, of the intrapulmonary pulmonary arteries).

Patients with pulmonary vascular disease constitute a large proportion of adult patients with congenital heart disease referred for

preoperative anesthesia evaluation and consultation before noncardiac surgery. These patients face significant perioperative risks, which can be greatly minimized by a physiologically appropriate anesthetic plan. Fixed pulmonary vascular resistance precludes rapid adaptation by the patient to intraoperative hemodynamic changes. Changes in the relative ratio of systemic to pulmonary vascular resistance are mirrored in the relative degree of right-to-left shunting. Close monitoring of intravascular volume and extremely cautious use of systemic vasodilators, including regional anesthesia, are mandatory. Epidural anesthesia has been used successfully in patients with pulmonary hypertension secondary to congenital heart disease, particularly during labor and delivery[68-71] and has been reported during other surgery.[72,73] It must be stressed that these reports remain anecdotal only at this time. If regional anesthesia is used, the following caveats would seem to apply. First, epidural anesthesia would seem to be safer than subarachnoid anesthesia, as the onset will be slower and the decrease in systemic vascular resistance can be managed more carefully. Second, if epidural anesthesia is used, the local anesthetic should be administered slowly and in small increments. Finally, it is likely that appropriate thoracic epidural anesthesia would have less of an effect altering the normal balance of systemic and pulmonary vascular resistances. Postoperative postural hypotension can significantly increase the degree of right-to-left shunting, and postoperative patients should change position slowly.

Placement of a pulmonary arterial catheter is in itself problematic and not without risk in patients with pulmonary arterial hypertension as well as the hemostatic abnormalities of congenital heart disease.[74] Both abnormal intracardiac anatomy and right-to-left intracardiac shunting may make placement of a flow-directed catheter difficult if not impossible without the aid of fluoroscopy. In addition, information available from these catheters may not be needed, and the numbers supplied may be incorrect. Relative resistances in the pulmonary and systemic circulations are reflected rather directly by changes in systemic arterial saturation, which can be monitored continuously by pulse oximetry. Increases in systemic vascular resistance or decreases in pulmonary vascular resistance will be marked by increases in systemic oxygen saturation as pulmonary blood flow increases and the pulmonary to systemic blood flow ratio (Qp to Qs) increases. The reverse changes in resistances will be marked by decreases in oxygen saturation. Cardiac output measured by thermodilution will be inaccurate due to the intracardiac shunt. In addition, it is extremely unlikely that acute right ventricular failure will develop, as the intracardiac defect serves as a popoff to relieve pressure on the right side of the heart. The potential exception to this is the patient with single-ventricle physiology who may have poor preoperative ventricular function, as well as patients with atrial septal defects and pulmonary vascular disease who are capable of developing suprasystemic pulmonary arterial pressure and right ventricular failure.[75]

Fixed pulmonary vascular resistance is, by definition, unresponsive to pharmacological intervention. Nevertheless, it would seem prudent to attempt to avoid factors known to increase pulmonary vascular resistance. These include cold, acidosis, hypercarbia, and hypoxia (in addition to preexistent hypoxemia). α-Adrenergic agents can increase pulmonary vascular resistance. However, it is typical that giving catecholamines with primary α-adrenergic effects, such as phenylephrine, increase pulmonary blood flow and, hence, systemic arterial oxygen saturation, by a more predominant effect in elevating systemic vascular resistance. Hypovolemia and systemic vasodilation both increase right-to-left shunt.

Appropriate nerve blocks offer an attractive alternative to general or major neuraxial anesthesia. If general anesthesia cannot be avoided, serious consideration should be given to returning the patient to the postanesthesia care unit (PACU) or an ICU, with the trachea still intubated and with plans for gradual recovery from anesthesia and extubation several hours later. Because of the high risk, after major surgery one should plan to observe these patients overnight in an ICU or monitored observation unit, depending on the facilities available. Clearly, this decision will be based on several factors, including the length and severity of the surgery, the patient's baseline hemodynamic status, and prior experience anesthetizing the patient for noncardiac surgery, if there was any. After an appropriate PACU stay, same-day discharge to home is appropriate after uncomplicated minor surgical procedures.

PERIOPERATIVE ISSUES

Social Issues

Most adults with congenital heart disease lead functional, productive lives. The Second Natural History Study of Congenital Heart Disease[76] showed that, overall, such patients were well-educated and productive members of society. However, a Finnish study found that these patients were more prone to have a dependent life-style; they lived with their parents and were more likely to be unmarried.[77] This was particularly true for the patients with cyanotic disease.

Another issue of major potential impact for young patients with congenital heart disease as they reach the age of majority is that they will no longer qualify for health insurance under either their parents' policy or under crippled children's services.[78] Presently, more than one-half are denied health insurance in whole or in part due to pre-existing conditions.[79]

Preoperative Medication

There is no contraindication to appropriate preoperative sedation in adults with congenital heart disease, either cyanotic or acyanotic, in the absence of severely depressed ventricular function. In fact, patients with unpalliated tetralogy of Fallot or pulmonary vascular disease would be particularly well-served by adequate preoperative anxiolysis. Many of these patients will be receiving digoxin as an inotrope, or diuretics, on a chronic basis. If the surgical procedure will involve manipulation of the heart, either by the surgeon or by placement of intracardiac catheters, it is our practice to withhold digoxin on the morning of surgery. Morning digoxin will result in peak myocardial digoxin levels at about the time the heart is stimulated, and it is our experience that there is an increased incidence of arrhythmias in this circumstance with direct cardiac stimulation. Should additional intraoperative inotropy be required, there are a variety of intravenous inotropic agents available, all of which are far more potent inotropes than digoxin. However, patients receiving digoxin for arrhythmia control should continue digoxin until surgery. Diuretics are probably best held on the morning of surgery to ensure adequate intravascular volume at the time of induction of anesthesia. Other cardiac medications are routinely continued until the time of surgery.

Vascular Access

Individual patients may have abnormalities that may restrict placement of arterial or venous catheters or may introduce artifacts into the pressures reflected by these catheters. These are summarized in Table 8–4. Impeded access to the right atrium from the femoral veins

TABLE 8–4. VASCULAR ACCESS CONSIDERATIONS

Femoral vein thrombosis or ligation after catheterization
Discontinuity of inferior vena cava and right atrium
Reduced lower extremity blood pressure with coarctation
Discontinuity of subclavian artery with classic Blalock-Taussig anastomosis
Stenosis at anastomotic site with modified Blalock-Taussig anastomosis
Artifactually elevated right arm blood pressure with supravalvar aortic stenosis
Risk of catheter-related thrombosis of superior vena cava catheters with Glenn or
    Fontan procedures
Risk of paradoxical air emboli

may not allow passage of long femoral venous catheters. There may be thrombosis of one or both femoral veins consequent to prior cardiac catheterizations. Vein obstruction is particularly common after passage of a relatively large balloon septostomy (Rashkind) catheter in the newborn period and is likely to be more common after introduction of other various interventional catheters, which tend to be fairly large in diameter. Cardiac catheterization, even in the smallest infants, has typically been done percutaneously for the past 2 decades. However, patients who had catheterizations prior to that time may likely have had them done by means of a cutdown. The cutdown may have been done to the saphenous vein or the femoral vein, and the vein may have been repaired or ligated. These data will not be apparent unless the original catheterization report is reviewed.

Patients with visceral heterotaxy and polysplenia typically have an interrupted inferior vena cava with venous return continuing via the hemiazygous vein (azygous continuation), making passage of a long catheter from the inferior vena cava to the right atrium in the operating room difficult, if not impossible. Short femoral venous catheters can, however, be introduced into these patients. It is preferable to avoid catheterizing the superior vena cava via the internal jugular or subclavian veins in patients who have had a Glenn anastomosis (superior vena cava to pulmonary artery) or a Fontan procedure done by means of a lateral tunnel approach, particularly if the catheter is to remain in situ for some time postoperatively. Catheter-related thrombosis of the superior vena cava, although rare, can be catastrophic in these patients.

Due to the risk of air emboli, strict attention must be paid to ensuring that all intravenous lines remain free of air bubbles. This is not only true in patients with obvious right-to-left shunts but also in patients with intracardiac shunts with the potential for right-to-left shunting. For example, there is the potential for right-to-left shunting in the presence of an atrial septal defect or patent foramen ovale with increased intrathoracic pressure.[80] Air and particle filters are commercially available but are inadequate for rapid infusions of fluid in adults. It has been recommended in the past that, in cases in which the inadvertent injection of small air bubbles would be a problem, that drugs be injected into a rubber injection port, avoiding the small bubbles that inexorably accumulate in stopcocks. That recommendation would appear to be inappropriate in the current needleless environment, and all syringes should be briefly and gently aspirated before injection to clear any bubble from the stopcock.

Arterial access may also be compromised. Residual aortic coarctation or recoarctation makes pressures proximal to the coarctation higher than those that are distal. Patients with a classic Blalock-Taussig anastomosis have discontinuity of the subclavian artery, typically with absent brachial-radial pulses in the affected arm, although pulses, occasionally strong, may be palpated. Blood pressure should be monitored in the opposite arm. Patients who have had bilateral Blalock-Taussig anastomoses should have arterial pressure monitored in a lower extremity. Even though the modified Blalock-Taussig anastomosis, which uses a synthetic anastomosis between the subclavian and pulmonary arteries, preserves continuity of the subclavian artery, there may be partial obstruction at the site of the anastomosis. Blood pressure should be obtained in the opposite arm, or the accuracy of the blood pressure on the side of the shunt should be confirmed preoperatively by comparing pressures obtained in each arm. Patients with supravalvar aortic stenosis may have elevated systolic blood pressure in the right arm, which is known as the Coanda effect.[81,82]

INFECTIVE ENDOCARDITIS PROPHYLAXIS

The clinical setting of endocarditis has changed over the past several decades with the introduction of intracardiac surgery, prosthetic devices, indwelling catheters, and hyperalimentation.[83] Endocarditis may occur years after cardiac surgical repair and may involve atypical organisms.[84] There are two major etiological factors in the development of endocarditis, namely, a susceptible cardiac or vascular lesion and a source for bacteremia. Lesions at risk are marked by high-velocity flow, jet impact, and local increases in shear rate. Among the congenital lesions, the lesions at greatest risk for the development of endocarditis in the adult are bicuspid aortic valve, restrictive ventricular septal defect, tetralogy of Fallot, high-pressure atrioventricular valve regurgitation, and aortic valve regurgitation. Prior surgical intervention may have had a significant effect on the risk of developing endocarditis. Certain procedures, ligation of a patent ductus arteriosus as an example, eliminate the risk, whereas others, prosthetic valves or conduits, for example, increase the risk.

A list of conditions requiring, or not requiring, antibiotic prophylaxis, is shown in Table 8–5. Not all operations or invasive procedures result in bacteremia, and thus not all require antibiotic prophylaxis. A partial list of procedures not requiring prophylaxis is given in Table 8–5. A complete guide to endocarditis prophylaxis is published by the American Heart Association.[85] Of note, orotracheal intubation is unassociated with bacteremia, but passage of catheters transnasally is.[86,87] Transesophageal echocardiography results in an extremely low risk for the development of endocarditis, with or without the use of antibiotic

TABLE 8–5. ENDOCARDITIS PROPHYLAXIS WITH ANTIBIOTICS

Some conditions requiring endocarditis prophylaxis
Prosthetic valves (both bioprosthetic and homograft)
Previous bacterial endocarditis
Systemic-pulmonary shunts (e.g., Blalock-Taussig)
Conditions not requiring prophylaxis
Isolated secundum atrial septal defect
Surgical repair beyond 6 months without residua of secundum atrial septal defect, ventricular septal defect, or patent ductus arteriosus
Some procedures not requiring prophylaxis
Injection of intraoral anesthetics
Tympanostomy tube placement
Orotracheal intubation
Flexible bronchoscopy with or without biopsy
Cardiac catheterization
Endoscopy with or without biopsy
Transesophageal echocardiography
Cesarean section
In the absence of infection: urethral catheterization, dilation and curettage, uncomplicated vaginal delivery, therapeutic abortion, sterilization procedures, insertion and removal of intrauterine devices

prophylaxis.[88] Unfortunately, bacterial endocarditis may not be uniformly prevented by antibiotic prophylaxis.[89,90]

INDUCTION AND MAINTENANCE OF ANESTHESIA

A wide variety of anesthetic agents have been used to induce and maintain anesthesia in patients with congenital heart disease. It is assumed that the reader is aware of the various hemodynamic effects of the available agents. Space does not permit even a partial discussion of the most appropriate regimen for each of the possible permutations of anesthetic agent and congenital lesion. Anesthesia for each of the most important lesions is discussed in the appropriate section of the major anesthesia texts or in subspecialty texts, such as that edited by Lake.[11] Clearly, the appropriate anesthetic technique is dictated by the relevant physiology, which can only be fully understood by a complete review of the history, physical examination, and relevant laboratory data.

Patients typically receive supplemental oxygen during induction of anesthesia. A minimal increase of systemic oxygen tension in response to supplemental oxygen is a hallmark of cyanosis due to cardiac disease.[91] Patients with desaturation due to pulmonary edema or to cyanotic lesions, which have both increased pulmonary blood flow and right-to-left shunts (truncus arteriosus or unobstructed total anomalous pulmonary venous return, for example) can manifest systemic oxygen tension exceeding 150 mm Hg in response to an F_{IO_2} of 1.0, but these circumstances would be exceedingly rare in the adult population. The physiologic effects of agents used to induce and maintain anesthesia may be complimentary or opposite. For example, following induction of anesthesia in cyanotic patients with a wide variety of agents, systemic oxygen saturation can be expected to increase.[92] Although the vasodilatory effects of these agents would be expected to increase the degree of right-to-left shunting and decrease systemic arterial oxygen saturation, presumably this effect is more than offset by the decrease in oxygen consumption accompanying anesthesia. As a result, mixed venous oxygen saturation is increased, with a subsequent increase in systemic oxygen saturation after shunting of this blood to the systemic circulation.

The negative inotropic effects inherent in the volatile agents in particular would be expected to be of benefit in lesions marked by dynamic obstruction to ventricular emptying, such as tetralogy of Fallot. Dynamic obstruction is also frequently encountered with D-transposition of the great arteries and single ventricle of the left ventricular type.

In adults, nitrous oxide has been reported to decrease cardiac output[93,94] and systemic arterial pressure. Perhaps more importantly, it has been reported to increase pulmonary vascular resistance, particularly in patients in whom the pulmonary vascular resistance is already elevated,[95-97] clearly problematic in patients with already elevated pulmonary vascular resistance or in those who require a very low resistance, for example patients after undergoing the Glenn or Fontan procedures. However, in children no increase in pulmonary vascular resistance was seen with 50% nitrous oxide, regardless of preexistent pulmonary vascular resistance.[98] Nitrous oxide and halothane are routinely used to induce anesthesia in cyanotic pediatric patients, and systemic oxygen saturation routinely increases at this time,[92,99] suggesting that if nitrous oxide does increase pulmonary vascular resistance, this effect must be very small. Although nitrous oxide use precludes the use of 100% oxygen, these patients will still be receiving greater than the F_{IO_2} of 0.21 that they usually breathe. In addition, decrements in F_{IO_2} have only minimal effects on systemic arterial oxygenation when desaturation is due to right-to-left shunting.[91] One caution regarding the use of nitrous oxide in patients with right-to-left shunts is the possibility of nitrous oxide to expand a surgically introduced air embolus. Nitrous oxide should probably be used cautiously, if at all, in patients with intracardiac shunts who are having surgical procedures at risk for introducing air emboli.

For patients with large left-to-right shunts at the ventricular or great vessel level, moderate hypercarbia and minimizing FiO_2 will increase pulmonary blood flow and decrease the amount of shunting, in turn decreasing the left ventricular diastolic volume and improving the ventricular oxygen supply-demand relationship. It is likely, though, that patients with excessive pulmonary blood flow will have developed adequate elevation in pulmonary vascular resistance to self-limit excessive flows by adulthood.

Neuraxial blockade would be expected to be relatively contraindicated in patients requiring maintenance of systemic vascular resistance; however, several groups have reported very cautious use of epidural anesthesia in a very few patients with pulmonary arterial hypertension[72,73] and continuous spinal anesthesia with valval aortic stenosis.[100] Clearly, the choice to use neuraxial blockade in these patients requires at the least that the anesthetic be given slowly, incrementally, and with appropriate monitoring.

POSTOPERATIVE MANAGEMENT

Clearly, these patients require close observation in the PACU. No specific duration of observation can be generalized, as this depends on the underlying disease and the operation done. Patients with good preexisting hemodynamic function with minor noncardiac surgery can be treated as would any other patient and are not excluded from ambulatory surgery. As discussed above, patients with cyanotic disease will benefit little, if at all, from increased inspired oxygen, a response that should be made known to the nurses caring for the patient so as to avoid needless prolonged courses of supplemental oxygen and delayed transfer from the PACU. Hypovolemia develops not infrequently, sometimes insidiously, in the postoperative patient. In many patients with cyanotic heart disease this will result in increased right-to-left shunting with worsening cyanosis. Cyanotic, erythrocytotic patients should have serial hematocrits followed after any procedure that has resulted in significant blood loss, and a hematocrit approximating the preoperative level should be maintained postoperatively.

The presence of cyanotic congenital heart disease does not exclude in any way appropriate postoperative pain control, including the appropriate use of narcotics. These patients have an essentially normal ventilatory response to hypercarbia and may be given normal doses of parenteral, intrathecal, or epidural narcotics. Patients with labile pulmonary hypertension in particular will benefit from good postoperative analgesia. Analgesics that decrease systemic vascular resistance should be used with caution in patients with Eisenmenger physiology or uncorrected tetralogy of Fallot.

Should patients who have had a Glenn or Fontan procedure require postoperative ventilation, an effort should be made to minimize pulmonary artery pressure by limiting positive inspiratory pressure and to optimize functional residual capacity by the judicious use of low levels of positive end-expiratory pressure (PEEP).

CONCLUSION

Adult patients presenting with congenital heart disease are an extremely disparate group and represent a large variety of pathophysiologies. Because of this, patients should have preoperative anesthetic evaluation scheduled far enough in advance of surgery to allow for adequate retrieval and review of all appropriate laboratory data, as well as time to obtain consultation, if necessary. This is most efficiently done in large centers with an already existing adult congenital heart disease center. In such centers it is most useful if one, or at least a very small number, of anesthesiologists be either consultants to the adult congenital heart disease center or, better yet, be a member of the center. These individuals can be much help in providing simplified access to the preanesthetic evaluation process. They may elect to administer the anesthetic personally or may elect to have another member of the anesthesia staff do it after written and/or verbal consultation. It has been our experience that in many cases the concerns regarding whether to schedule (or to cancel) a proposed noncardiac surgical procedure in adults with congenital heart disease revolve around perioperative anesthetic issues and not around surgical issues. Appropriate, well thought out preanesthetic discussions with patients and surgeons can often help plan for a safe anesthetic for procedures that might have been rejected out of hand by noncardiac surgeons with only a limited knowledge of congenital heart disease.

References

1. Moller JH, Anderson RC: 1,000 consecutive children with a cardiac malformation with 26- to 37-year follow-up. Am J Cardiol 70:661–667, 1992
2. Perloff JK: Medical center experiences. J Am Coll Cardiol 18:315–318, 1991
3. Morris CD, Menashe VD: Twenty-five-year mortality after surgical repair of congenital heart defect in childhood. A population-based cohort study. JAMA 266:3447–3452, 1991

4. Hoffman JI, Christianson R: Congenital heart disease in a cohort of 19,502 births with long-term follow-up. Am J Cardiol 42:641–647, 1978
5. Manning JA: Insurability and employability of young cardiac patients. Cardiovasc Clin 11:117–127, 1981
6. Mahoney LT, Skorton DJ: Insurability and employability. J Am Coll Cardiol 18:334–336, 1991
7. Morris CD, Menashe VD: Twenty-five-year mortality after surgical repair of congenital heart defect in childhood: A population-based cohort study. JAMA 266:3447–3452, 1991
8. Emmanouilides GC, Riemenschneider TA, Allen HD, Gutgesell HP (eds): Moss' Heart Disease in Infants, Children, and Adolescents. Baltimore, Williams & Wilkins, 1995
9. Rudolph AM: Congenital Diseases of the Heart. Chicago, Yearbook Medical Publishers, 1974
10. Fyler, DC (ed): Nadas' Pediatric Cardiology. Philadelphia, Hanley and Belfus, 1992
11. Lake CA (ed): Pediatric Cardiac Anesthesia. Norwalk, CT, Appleton & Lange, 1993
12. Kamba J: Cardiac Anesthesia for Infants and Children. St. Louis, Mosby, 1994
13. Mitchell SC, Korones SB, Berendes HW: Congenital heart disease in 56,109 births: Incidence and natural history. Circulation 43:323–332, 1971
14. Campbell M: Natural history of coarctation of the aorta. Br Heart J 32:663–640, 1970
15. Baum VC: The adult with congenital heart disease. J Cardiothorac Vasc Anesth, in press, 1996
16. Roberts WC (ed): Adult Congenital Heart Disease. Philadelphia, FA Davis, 1987
17. Engle MA, Perloff JK (eds): Congenital Heart Disease after Surgery: Benefits, Residua, Sequelae. New York, Yorke, 1983
18. Wooley CF, Sparks EH: Congenital heart disease, heritable cardiovascular disease, and pregnancy. Prog Cardiovasc Dis 35:41–60, 1992
19. Pitkin RM, Perloff JK, Koos BJ, Beall MH: Pregnancy and congenital heart disease. Ann Intern Med 112:445–454, 1990
20. Elkayam U, Gleicher N: Cardiac Problems in Pregnancy: Diagnosis and Management of Maternal and Fetal Disease. New York, Alan R. Liss, 1990
21. Presbitero P, Somerville J, Stone S, Aruta E, Spiegelhalter D, Rabajoli F: Pregnancy in cyanotic congenital heart disease: Outcome of mother and fetus. Circulation 89:2673–2676, 1994
22. Graham TP: Ventricular performance in congenital heart disease. Circulation 84:2259–2274, 1991
23. Mendelson MA: Pregnancy in the woman with congenital heart disease. Am J Cardiac Imaging 9:44–52, 1995
24. Bancalari E, Jesse MJ, Gelband H, Garcia O: Lung mechanics in congenital heart disease with increased and decreased pulmonary blood flow. J Pediatr 90:192–195, 1977
25. Pande JN, Gupta SP, Guleria JS: Ventilatory response to inhaled CO_2 at high altitude. Respiration 31:473–483, 1974
26. Sietsema KE, Perloff JK: Cyanotic congenital heart disease: Dynamics of oxygen uptake and control of ventilation during exercise. In Perloff JK, Child JS (eds): Congenital Heart Disease in Adults, pp. 104–110. Philadelphia, WB Saunders, 1991

27. Sorensen SC, Severinghaus JW: Respiratory insensitivity to acute hypoxia persisting after correction of tetralogy of Fallot. J Appl Physiol 25: 221–223, 1968
28. Edelmann NH, Lahiri S, Braudo L, Cherniak NS, Fishman AP: The ventilatory response to hypoxia in cyanotic congenital heart disease. N Engl J Med 282:405–411, 1970
29. Blesa MI, Lahiri S, Rashkind WJ, Fishman AP: Normalization of the blunted ventilatory response to acute hypoxia in congenital cyanotic heart disease. N Engl J Med 296:237–241, 1977
30. Burrows FA: Physiologic dead space, venous admixture, and the arterial to end-tidal carbon dioxide difference in infants and children undergoing cardiac surgery. Anesthesiology 70:219–225, 1989
31. Stanger P, Lucas RV, Edwards JE: Anatomic factors causing respiratory distress in acyanotic congenital cardiac disease: Special reference to bronchial obstruction. Pediatrics 43:760–769, 1969
32. Aboussouan LS, O'Donovan PB, Moodie DS, Gragg LA, Stoller JK: Hypoplastic trachea in Down's syndrome. Am Rev Respir Dis 147:72–75, 1993
33. Roth A, Rosenthal A, Hall JE, Mizel M: Scoliosis and congenital heart disease. Clin Orthop 93:95–102, 1973
34. Moore JW, Kirby WC, Madden WA, Gaither NS: Development of pulmonary arteriovenous malformations after modified Fontan operations. J Thorac Cardiovasc Surg 98:1045–1050, 1989
35. Bernstein HS, Brook MM, Silverman NH, Bristow J: Early development of pulmonary arteriovenous fistulae in children following cavopulmonary shunt (abstr). Circulation 90 (suppl I):I-421, 1994
36. Humes RA, Mair DD, Porter CB, Puga FJ, Schaff HV, Danielson GK: Results of the modified Fontan operation in adults. Am J Cardiol 61: 602–604, 1988
37. Rosove MH, Perloff JK, Hocking WG, Child JS, Canobbio MM, Skorton DJ: Chronic hypoxaemia and decompensated erythrocytosis in cyanotic congenital heart disease. Lancet 2:313–315, 1986
38. Berman WJ, Wood SC, Yabek SM, Dillon T, Fripp RR, Burstein R: Systemic oxygen transport in patients with congenital heart disease. Circulation 75:360–368, 1987
39. Perloff JK, Rosove MH, Child JS, Wright GB: Adults with cyanotic congenital heart disease: Hematologic management. Ann Intern Med 109: 406–413, 1988
40. Rosenthal A, Nathan DG, Marty AT, Button LN, Miettinen OS, Nadas AS: Acute hemodynamic effects of red cell volume reduction in polycythemia of cyanotic congenital heart disease. Circulation 42:297–308, 1970
41. Oldershaw PJ, Sutton MG: Haemodynamic effects of haematocrit reduction in patients with polycythaemia secondary to cyanotic congenital heart disease. Br Heart J 44:584–588, 1980
42. Schmid-Schonbein H, Wells R, Goldstone J: Influence of deformability of human red cells upon blood viscosity. Circ Res 25:131–143, 1969
43. Linderkamp O, Klose HJ, Betke K et al: Increased blood viscosity in patients with cyanotic congenital heart disease and iron deficiency. J Pediatr 95:567–569, 1979
44. Gidding SS, Stockman JA: Effect of iron deficiency on tissue oxygen delivery in cyanotic congenital heart disease. Am J Cardiol 61:605–607, 1988

45. England JM, Walford DM, Waters DA: Re-assessment of the reliability of the haematocrit. Br J Haematol 23:247–256, 1972
46. Territo MC, Rosove MH, Perloff JK: Cyanotic congenital heart disease: Hematologic management, renal function and urate metabolism. In Perloff JK, Child JS (eds): Congenital Heart Disease in Adults, pp. 93–103. Philadelphia, WB Saunders, 1991
47. Bhargava M, Sanyal SK, Thapar MK, Kumar S, Hooja V: Impairment of platelet adhesiveness and platelet factor 3 activity in cyanotic congenital heart disease. Acta Haematol 55:216–223, 1976
48. Ekert H, Dowling SV: Platelet release abnormality and reduced prothrombin levels in children with cyanotic congenital heart disease. Aust Paediatr J 13:17–21, 1977
49. Mauer HM, McCue CM, Caul J, Still WJ: Impairment in platelet aggregation in congenital heart disease. Blood 40:207–216, 1972
50. Ware JA, Reaves WH, Horak JK, Solis RT: Defective platelet aggregation in patients undergoing surgical repair of cyanotic congenital heart disease. Ann Thorac Surg 36:289–294, 1983
51. Colon-Otero G, Gilchrist GS, Holcomb GR, Ilstrup DM, Bowie EJ: Preoperative evaluation of hemostasis in patients with congenital heart disease. Mayo Clin Proc 62:379–385, 1987
52. Ekert H, Gilchrist GS, Stanton R, Hammond D: Hemostasis in cyanotic congenital heart disease. J Pediatr 76:221–230, 1970
53. Suarez CR, Menendez CE, Griffin AJ, Ow EP, Walenga JM, Fareed J: Cyanotic congenital heart disease in children: Hemostatic disorders and relevance of molecular markers of hemostasis. Semin Thromb Hemost 10:285–289, 1984
54. Wedemeyer AL, Edson JR, Krivit W: Coagulation in cyanotic congenital heart disease. Am J Dis Child 124:656–660, 1972
55. Rosove MH, Hocking WG, Harwig SS, Perloff JK: Studies of beta-thromboglobulin, platelet factor 4, and fibrinopeptide A in erythrocytosis due to cyanotic congenital heart disease. Thromb Res 29:225–235, 1983
56. Gill JC, Wilson AD, Endres-Brooks J, Montgomery RR: Loss of the largest von Willebrand factor multimers from the plasma of patients with congenital cardiac defects. Blood 67:758–761, 1986
57. Weinstein M, Ware JA, Troll J, Salzman E: Changes in von Willebrand factor during cardiac surgery: Effect of desmopressin acetate. Blood 71:1648–1655, 1988
58. Spear GS: The glomerular lesion of cyanotic congenital heart disease. Johns Hopkins Med J 140:185–188, 1977
59. Ross EA, Perloff JK, Danovitch GM, Child JS, Canobbio MM: Renal function and urate metabolism in late survivors with cyanotic congenital heart disease. Circulation 73:396–400, 1986
60. Young D: Hyperuricemia in cyanotic congenital heart disease [Letter]. Am J Dis Child 134:902–903, 1980
61. Perloff JK, Marelli A: Neurological and psychosocial disorders in adults with congenital heart disease. Heart Dis Stroke 1:218–224, 1992
62. Perloff JK, Marelli AJ, Miner PD: Risk of stroke in adults with cyanotic congenital heart disease. Circulation 87:1954–1959, 1993
63. Simon AB, Zloto AE: Coarctation of the aorta. Longitudinal assessment of operated patients. Circulation 50:456–464, 1974
64. Kurlan R, Krall RL, Deweese JA: Vertebrobasilar ischemia after total repair of tetralogy of Fallot: Significance of subclavian steal created by Blalock-Taussig anastomosis. Stroke 15:359–362, 1984

65. Corone S, Davido A, Lang T, Corone P: Outcome of patients with Eisenmenger syndrome: Apropos of 62 cases followed-up for an average of 16 years. Arch Mal Coeur Vaiss 85:521–526, 1992

66. Heath D, Edwards JE: The pathology of pulmonary vascular disease. Circulation 18:533–547, 1958

67. Rabinovitch M, Haworth SG, Castaneda AR, Nadas AS, Reid L: Lung biopsy in congenital heart disease: A morphometric approach to pulmonary vascular disease. Circulation 58:1107–1122, 1978

68. Smedstad KG, Cramb R, Morison DH: Pulmonary hypertension and pregnancy: A series of eight cases. Can J Anaesth 41:502–512, 1994

69. Atanassoff PG, Schmid ER, Jenni R, Arbenz U, Alon E, Pasch T: Epidural anesthesia for a cesarean section in a patient with pulmonary atresia and ventricular septal defect. J Clin Anesth 3:399–402, 1991

70. Breen TW, Janzen JA: Pulmonary hypertension and cardiomyopathy: Anaesthetic management for caesarean section. Can J Anaesth 38:895–899, 1991

71. Spinnato JA, Kraynack BJ, Cooper MW: Eisenmenger's syndrome in pregnancy: Epidural anesthesia for elective cesarean section. N Engl J Med 304:1215–1217, 1981

72. Selsby DS, Sugden JC: Epidural anaesthesia for bilateral inguinal herniorrhaphy in Eisenmenger's syndrome. Anaesthesia 44:130–132, 1989

73. Mallampati SR: Low thoracic epidural anaesthesia for elective cholecystectomy in a patient with congenital heart disease and pulmonary hypertension. Can Anaesth Soc J 30:72–76, 1983

74. Devitt JH, Noble WH, Byrick RJ: A Swan-Ganz catheter related complication in a patient with Eisenmenger's syndrome. Anesthesiology 57:335–337, 1982

75. Perloff JK: The Clinical Recognition of Congenital Heart Disease. Philadelphia, WB Saunders, 1987

76. O'Fallon WM, Weidman WH: Long-term follow-up of congenital aortic stenosis, pulmonary stenosis and ventricular septal defect. Circulation 87(suppl I):I1–I126, 1995

77. Kokkonen J, Paavilainen T: Social adaptation of young adults with congenital heart disease. Int J Cardiol 36:23–29, 1992

78. Allen HD, Gersony WM, Taubert KA: Insurability of the adolescent and young adult with heart disease: Report from the Fifth Conference on Insurability, October 3–4, 1991, Columbus, Ohio. Circulation 86:703–710, 1992

79. Truesdell SC, Clark EB: Health insurance status in a cohort of children and young adults with congenital cardiac diagnoses (abstr). Circulation 84(suppl 2):II386, 1991

80. Jaffe RA, Pinto FJ, Schnittger I, Siegel LC, Wranne B, Brock-Utne JG: Aspects of mechanical ventilation affecting interatrial shunt flow during general anesthesia. Anesth Analg 75:484–488, 1992

81. French JW, Guntheroth WG: An explanation of asymmetric upper extremity blood pressures in supravalvular aortic stenosis: The Coanda effect. Circulation 42:31–36, 1970

82. Goldstein RE, Epstein SE: Mechanism of elevated innominate artery pressures in supravalvular aortic stenosis. Circulation 42:23–29, 1970

83. Child JS, Perloff JK: Infective endocarditis: Risks and prophylaxis. In Perloff JK, Child JS (eds): Congenital Heart Disease in Adults, pp. 111–123. Philadelphia, WB Saunders, 1991

84. Saleh MA, Al-Madan MS, Erwa HH, Sohel SZ, Sanyal SK: First case of human infection caused by *Pasteurella gallinarum* causing infective en-

docarditis in an adolescent 10 years after surgical correction for truncus arteriosus. Pediatrics 944–948, 1995

85. Dajani AS, Bisno AL, Chung KJ et al: Prevention of bacterial endocarditis: Recommendations by the American Heart Association. JAMA 264: 2919–2922, 1990

86. Berry FA, Blankenbaker WL, Ball CG: Comparison of bacteremia occurring with nasotracheal and orotracheal intubation. Anesth Analg 52: 873–876, 1973

87. LeFrock JL, Klainer AS, Wu WH, Turndorf H: Transient bacteremia associated with nasotracheal suctioning. JAMA 236:1610–1611, 1976

88. Mentec H, Vignon P, Terre S et al: Frequency of bacteremia associated with transesophageal echocardiography in intensive care unit patients: A prospective study of 139 patients. Crit Care Med 23:1194–1199, 1995

89. Durack DT: Prevention of infective endocarditis. N Engl J Med 332:38–44, 1995

90. Van der Meer JT, Van Wijk W, Thompson J, Vandenbroucke JP, Valkenburg HA, Michel MF: Efficacy of antibiotic prophylaxis for prevention of native-valve endocarditis. Lancet 339:135–139, 1992

91. Lawler PG, Nunn JF: A reassessment of the validity of the iso-shunt graph. Br J Anaesth 56:1325–1335, 1984

92. Laishley RS, Burrows FA, Lerman J, Roy WL: Effect of anesthetic induction regimens on oxygen saturation in cyanotic congenital heart disease. Anesthesiology 65:673–677, 1986

93. Siker D, Pagel PS, Pelc LR, Schmeling WT, Warltier DC: Nitrous oxide impairs functional recovery of stunned myocardium in barbiturate-anesthetized, acutely instrumented dogs. Anesth Analg 75:539–548, 1992

94. Messina AG, Yao FS, Canning H et al: The effect of nitrous oxide on left ventricular pump performance and contractility in patients with coronary artery disease: Effect of preoperative ejection fraction. Anesth Analg 77:954–962, 1993

95. Hilgenberg JC, McCammon RL, Stoelting RK: Pulmonary and systemic vascular responses to nitrous oxide in patients with mitral stenosis and pulmonary hypertension. Anesth Analg 59:323–326, 1980

96. Lappas DG, Buckley MJ, Laver MB, Daggett WM, Lowenstein E: Left ventricular performance and pulmonary circulation following addition of nitrous oxide to morphine during coronary-artery surgery. Anesthesiology 43:61–69, 1975

97. Schulte-Sasse U, Hess W, Tarnow J: Pulmonary vascular responses to nitrous oxide in patients with normal and high pulmonary vascular resistance. Anesthesiology 57:9–13, 1982

98. Hickey PR, Hansen DD, Strafford M, Thompson JE, Jonas RE, Mayer JE: Pulmonary and systemic hemodynamic effects of nitrous oxide in infants with normal and elevated pulmonary vascular resistance. Anesthesiology 65:374–378, 1986

99. Greeley WJ, Bushman GA, Davis DP, Reves JG: Comparative effects of halothane and ketamine on systemic arterial oxygen saturation in children with cyanotic heart disease. Anesthesiology 65:666–668, 1986

100. Collard CD, Eappen S, Lynch EP, Concepcion M: Continuous spinal anesthesia with invasive hemodynamic monitoring for surgical repair of the hip in two patients with severe aortic stenosis. Anesth Analg 81: 195–198, 1995

101. Webb GD, Burrows FA: The risks of noncardiac surgery. J Am Coll Cardiol 18:323–325, 1991

Index

Page numbers followed by *t* or *f* indicate tables or figures, respectively.